Advances in Cosmetic Dermatology

Editors

NEIL S. SADICK
NILS KRUEGER

DERMATOLOGIC CLINICS

www.derm.theclinics.com

Consulting Editor
BRUCE H. THIERS

January 2014 • Volume 32 • Number 1

ELSEVIER

1600 John F. Kennedy Boulevard • Suite 1800 • Philadelphia, Pennsylvania, 19103-2899

http://www.theclinics.com

DERMATOLOGIC CLINICS Volume 32, Number 1
January 2014 ISSN 0733-8635, ISBN-13: 978-0-323-26388-7

Editor: Joanne Husovski
Developmental Editor: Susan Showalter

Dermatologic Clinics (ISSN 0733-8635) is published quarterly by Elsevier Inc., 360 Park Avenue South, New York, NY 10010-1710. Months of publication are January, April, July, and October. Business and editorial offices: 1600 John F. Kennedy Blvd., Suite 1800, Philadelphia, PA 19103-2899. Customer service office: 11830 Westline Drive, St. Louis, MO 63146. Periodicals postage paid at New York, NY, and additional mailing offices. Subscription prices are USD 365.00 per year for US individuals, USD 559.00 per year for US institutions, USD 425.00 per year for Canadian individuals, USD 681.00 per year for Canadian institutions, USD 495.00 per year for international individuals, USD 681.00 per year for international institutions, USD 165.00 per year for US students/residents, and USD 240.00 per year for Canadian and international students/residents. International air speed delivery is included in all *Clinics* subscription prices. All prices are subject to change without notice. **POSTMASTER:** Send address changes to *Dermatologic Clinics*, Elsevier Health Sciences Division, Subscription Customer Service, 3251 Riverport Lane, Maryland Heights, MO 63043. **Customer Service: 1-800-654-2452 (U.S. and Canada); 314-447-8871 (outside U.S. and Canada). Fax: 314-447-8029. E-mail: journalscustomerservice-usa@elsevier.com (for print support); journalsonlinesupport-usa@elsevier.com (for online support).**

Reprints. For copies of 100 or more, of articles in this publication, please contact the Commercial Reprints Department, Elsevier Inc., 360 Park Avenue South, New York, New York 10010-1710. Tel.: 212-633-3874; Fax: 212-633-3820; Email: repritns@elsevier.com.

The *Dermatologic Clinics* is covered in *MEDLINE/PubMed (Index Medicus)*, *Current Contents/Clinical Medicine*, *Excerpta Medica*, *Chemical Abstracts*, and *ISI/BIOMED*.

Printed and bound by CPI Group (UK) Ltd, Croydon, CR0 4YY

Transferred to digital print 2012

Contributors

CONSULTING EDITOR

BRUCE H. THIERS, MD
Professor and Chairman, Department of
Dermatology and Dermatologic Surgery,
Medical University of South Carolina,
Charleston, South Carolina

EDITORS

NEIL S. SADICK, MD, FACP, FAACS
Sadick Research Group; Clinical Professor,
Department of Dermatology, Weill Cornell
Medical College, New York, New York

NILS KRUEGER, PhD
Sadick Research Group, New York, New York

AUTHORS

MURAD ALAM, MD, MSCI
Professor, Department of Dermatology,
Otolaryngology-Head and Neck Surgery;
Chief, Section of Cutaneous and Aesthetic
Surgery, Department of Surgery, Northwestern
University, Chicago, Illinois

**MACRENE ALEXIADES-ARMENAKAS, MD,
PhD**
Dermatology and Laser Surgery Center,
New York, New York; Assistant Clinical
Professor, Department of Dermatology, Yale
University School of Medicine, New Haven,
Connecticut

KAREN L. BEASLEY, MD, FAAD
Clinical Assistant Professor of Dermatology,
University of Maryland School of Medicine,
Baltimore; The Maryland Laser, Skin and Vein
Institute, Hunt Valley, Maryland

DIANE BERSON, MD
Associate Clinical Professor of Dermatology,
Weill Medical College of Cornell University,
New York-Presbyterian, New York, New York

ANDREW DORIZAS, MD
Sadick Research Group, New York, New York

SABRINA GUILLEN FABI, MD, FAAD, FAACS
Voluntary Clinical Professor in Medicine/
Dermatology, University of California,
Associate, Goldman, Butterwick, Fitzpatrick,
Groff, and Fabi, Cosmetic Laser Dermatology,
San Diego, California

REBECCA FITZGERALD, MD
Assistant Clinical Instructor, Division of
Dermatology, University of California,
Los Angeles (UCLA), Los Angeles, California

BRUCE E. KATZ, MD
Director, Juva Skin and Laser Center; Clinical
Professor, Mt. Sinai School of Medicine,
Director, Cosmetic Surgery and Laser Clinic,
Mt. Sinai Medical Center, New York, New York

NILS KRUEGER, PhD
Sadick Research Group, New York, New York

STEFANIE LUEBBERDING, PhD
Dermatology and Laser Surgery Center,
New York, New York

SARAH MALERICH, BS
Fourth Year Medical Student, Lake Erie
College of Osteopathic Medicine, Bradenton,
Florida

ANDREI I. METELITSA, MD, FRCPC
Co-Director, Institute for Skin Advancement,
Assistant Clinical Professor, University of
Calgary, Calgary, Alberta, Canada

KIRA MINKIS, MD, PhD
Department of Dermatology, Northwestern
University, Chicago, Illinois

BERNARD NUSBAUM, MD
Hair Transplant Institute Miami, Coral Gables,
Florida

MICHELLE E. PARK
Research Fellow, Department of Dermatology,
Weill Cornell Medical College, New York,
New York

PAUL T. ROSE, MD, JD
Hair Transplant Institute Miami, Coral Gables,
Florida

ANTHONY M. ROSSI, MD
Memorial Sloan Kettering Cancer Center, Weill
Cornell Medical College; Juva Skin and Laser
Center, New York, New York

ASHLEY G. RUBIN, MD
Resident Physician, Division of Dermatology,
University of California, Los Angeles (UCLA),
Los Angeles, California

NEIL S. SADICK, MD, FACP, FAACS
Sadick Research Group; Clinical Professor,
Department of Dermatology, Weill
Cornell Medical College, New York,
New York

ROBERT A. WEISS, MD, FAAD, FACPh
Clinical Associate Professor of Dermatology,
Director, University of Maryland School of
Medicine, Baltimore; Director, The Maryland
Laser, Skin and Vein Institute, Hunt Valley,
Maryland

JONATHAN H. ZIPPIN, MD, PhD
Assistant Professor of Dermatology,
Department of Dermatology, Weill
Cornell Medical College, New York,
New York

Contents

tattoo ink. Current research in the field of tattoo removal is focused on faster lasers and more effective targeting of tattoo pigment particles including picosecond laser devices, multi-pass treatments, dermal scatter reduction, application of imiquimod, and the use of microencapsulated tattoo ink.

The latest innovation to hair restoration surgery has been the introduction of a robotic system for harvesting grafts. This system uses the follicular unit extraction/follicular isolation technique method for harvesting follicular units, which is particularly well suited to the abilities of a robotic technology. The ARTAS system analyzes images of the donor area and then a dual-chamber needle and blunt dissecting punch are used to harvest the follicular units. The robotic technology is now being used in various locations around the world. This article discusses the use of the robotic system, its capabilities, and the advantages and disadvantages of the system.

DERMATOLOGIC CLINICS

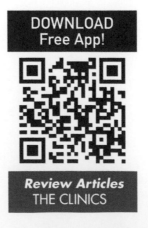

NOW AVAILABLE FOR YOUR iPhone and iPad

Erratum

In the October 2013 issue of Dermatologic Clinics, Dermoscopy, the name of the Author on the article Hair Shafts in Trichoscopy: Clues for Diagnosis of Hair and Scalp Diseases was misspelled. The correct spelling is Marta Kurzeja.

Dermatol Clin 32 (2014) ix
http://dx.doi.org/10.1016/j.det.2013.11.001

Preface
Cosmetic Dermatology

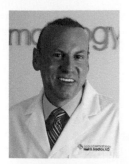
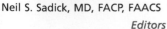
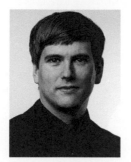

Neil S. Sadick, MD, FACP, FAACS   Nils Krueger, PhD

Editors

Cosmetic Dermatology plays a major role in physician practices nowadays. Patients' desire to stay young and attractive is no longer only influenced by living longer, but also by remaining longer in the workforce and being involved in longer or multiple interpersonal relationships during their life. However, modern patients are not willing to improve their appearance at any costs. They expect treatments and procedures to be effective but also, more importantly, to be safe and followed by minimum downtime. So-called "lunchtime procedures," which fit into busy schedules and come without downtime or side effects, are preferred nowadays by male and female patients that want to look fresh, but don't want others to know about their treatments.

Cosmetic Dermatology in the 21st century includes a broad spectrum of noninvasive and minimally invasive treatments and procedures including injectables like fillers and botulinum toxin products as well as devices that utilize light, radiofrequency, or ultrasound and robotic hair transplantations. All these modalities address typical signs of aging, such as wrinkles, skin laxity, discoloration, or hair loss, as well as aesthetic unpleasant body deformities including cellulite and localized fat deposits. Each technology can be used independently to treat a specific indication, but only when utilized in combination by an experienced dermatologist do they show their full potential. For state-of-the-art rejuvenation and body contouring, they should be used in a three-dimensional approach, which targets epidermal, dermal, and subcutaneous structures to achieve a complete global improvement in appearance.

The present volume of *Dermatology Clinics* presents articles in this regard and will hopefully give the practicing cosmetic dermatologists and cosmetic surgeons good insight of the emerging advances in this field.

Neil S. Sadick, MD, FACP, FAACS
Weill Cornell Medical College
Department of Dermatology
1300 York Avenue
New York, NY, USA

Nils Krueger, PhD
Sadick Research Group
911 Park Avenue
New York, NY 10075, USA

E-mail addresses:
nssderm@sadickdermatology.com (N.S. Sadick)
NKrueger@sadickdermatology.com (N. Krueger)

Dermatol Clin 32 (2014) xi
http://dx.doi.org/10.1016/j.det.2013.10.001
0733-8635/14/$ – see front matter

Allergic Contact Dermatitis to Cosmetics

Michelle E. Park*, Jonathan H. Zippin, MD, PhD*

KEYWORDS

- Cosmetic • Cosmetic allergy • Allergic contact dermatitis • ACD • Patch testing
- Cosmetic patch testing • Cosmetic series

KEY POINTS

- Cosmetics may cause allergic contact dermatitis (ACD) due to common allergenic components that are frequently found in cosmetics.
- The most common sites of reaction are the face and neck. The most common allergens in cosmetics are fragrances and preservatives.
- A thorough patient interview is the key to achieving proper diagnosis and management of cosmetic-induced ACD.
- Patch testing is the gold standard for diagnosing cosmetic-induced ACD, and the addition of a cosmetic series and testing of the patients' own products can be helpful.
- The mainstay of management is allergen avoidance.

INTRODUCTION

The history of cosmetic use is rich and antecedes written history, spanning civilizations and centuries that began with the ancient Egyptians using their natural resources to create a myriad of products such as scented oils, creams, lip stains, and eyeliners. Today, cosmetics are used worldwide and create a steadily increasing multibillion-dollar industry. The term "cosmetic", according to the US Food and Drug Administration (FDA), means "(1) articles intended to be rubbed, poured, sprinkled, sprayed on, introduced into, or otherwise applied to the human body or any part thereof for cleansing, beautifying, promoting attractiveness, or altering the appearance, and (2) articles intended for use as a component of any such articles; except that such term shall not include soap."[1] With a broad definition that encompasses facial makeup, skincare items, perfumes, hair and nail products, shaving gels or creams, and any personal hygiene product such as toothpaste or deodorant, efforts have been put in place by the creation of the Cosmetic Ingredient Review in 1976 and the FDA to moderate the safety of cosmetic products. However, it is estimated that an adverse reaction to cosmetics occurs approximately once every 13.3 years per person.[2] It is difficult to estimate the frequency of adverse reaction because cosmetics in the general population, and the prevalence is most likely underestimated due to most people do not seek medical advice and simply discontinue use of the product suspected of triggering a reaction.[3]

There are many types of adverse reactions caused by cosmetics. Most adverse reactions are irritant; however, type IV hypersensitivity, contact urticaria, photosensitization, pigmentary disorders, damage of hair and nails, paronychia, acneiform eruptions, folliculitis, and exacerbation of an established dermatosis may also occur.[4]

Conflict of Interest: None.

Department of Dermatology, Weill Cornell Medical College, 1305 York Avenue, 9th Floor, New York, NY 10021, USA

* Corresponding authors. Department of Dermatology, New York-Presbyterian Hospital, Weill Cornell Medical Center, 1305 York Avenue, 9th Floor, New York, NY 10021.

E-mail addresses: mip2038@med.cornell.edu; jhzippin@med.cornell.edu

Dermatol Clin 32 (2014) 1–11

http://dx.doi.org/10.1016/j.det.2013.09.006

0733-8635/14/$ – see front matter Published by Elsevier Inc.

Allergic contact dermatitis (ACD), or a type IV hypersensitivity reaction, is much less common than an irritant dermatitis, and several studies have found the prevalence of ACD to be less than 1% in the general population.[5–9] Type IV is a delayed-type hypersensitivity reaction that is T-cell mediated, wherein circulating or resident sensitized T cells are activated by the offending allergen to release pro-inflammatory cytokines. Sensitization depends on several factors including product composition, concentration of potential allergenic components, amount of product applied, application site, skin barrier integrity, and frequency and duration of application.[10,11] Sensitization usually requires repeated exposure and application to damaged skin.

EPIDEMIOLOGY

Although the prevalence of cosmetic allergy is found to be less than 1% in various studies, it is most likely an inaccurate number due to the tendency of patients to forgo seeking medical attention and discontinue use of the product on their own. A study conducted in the United States of patients with suspected ACD by the North American Contact Dermatitis Group (NACDG) found that after patch testing 10,061 patients over 7 years, 23.8% of female patients and 17.8% of male patients had at least one allergic patch-test reaction associated with a cosmetic source.[12] One review found the pooled prevalence rate of ACD to cosmetics in 7 different studies to be 9.8%.[13] The rate varies with time and geographic location, most influenced by the allergenicity of cosmetic ingredients, a population's increased use of cosmetics over time, and accessibility of allergens to be used in patch

testing.[14,15] Studies reporting the epidemiology of cosmetic allergy characterize the population most affected with cosmetic sensitivity as female between 20 and 55 years of age.[5–7]

EVALUATION

Cosmetic allergy occurs through direct application of an allergen, or the allergen can be airborne or transferred (usually from the hands and fingernails). **Table 1** lists the different ways in which an allergen may come in contact with the skin.

ACD can be considered in the differential diagnosis according to the site of the reaction on the body and the allergen most likely to come in contact with that region. There are certain areas of presentation where ACD should be considered because of their frequency of cosmetic contact and the possible allergens that such cosmetics contain. These areas are the face, eyelid, neck, hands, scalp, and anogenital region.

Patient evaluation should begin with a thorough medical history and careful investigation of products used by the patient in all settings (house and work), followed by a physical examination. A finding of dermatitis on the following areas should make the clinician suspicious of a cosmetic contact allergy.

FACE

The face is the most common site of ACD, and cosmetics are a common cause of this condition.[7,16] Because of the continually exposed nature of the face, cosmetic allergens come into contact with the face not only through direct application, but also indirectly through the air and through transfer from hands. A pattern of ACD on the face can appear patchy even when a product is applied to

Table 1
Modes of allergen transfer

Type	Definition	Example
Intentional direct contact	Allergenic ingredient in cosmetic product	Eye cosmetic, deodorant
Unintentional direct contact	Allergen-contaminated surface	Towel, pillow, telephone
Airborne	Gas, droplet, or particle in the atmosphere	Epoxy resin (occupation-related), cigarette smoke
Connubial	Contact with family, friends, colleagues	Perfume or hair dye from spouse
Ectopic	Transfer from one site of body to more sensitive area (ie, face, eyelids)	Fingernail varnish
Photosensitization	Photoallergens exposed to the sun	Photoallergens in sunscreen

the whole face. Facial contact dermatitis is most often thought to be bilateral, but clinicians must still consider this diagnosis even if the whole face is not involved. Of note, dermatitis involving the lateral face, forehead, eyelids, ears, and neck can be observed in patients that experience application of an allergen to the scalp that runs into these adjacent areas, creating a "rinse-off" pattern.[17]

Sometimes an offending agent is not obvious, such as when a patient is sensitized to allergens in cosmetic tools such as the rubber in cosmetic sponges.[18,19] Less obvious is when a cosmetic allergen has been transferred to a surface otherwise considered innocuous, such as a towel or telephone. The patient history is very important in determining the cause of allergy in such cases.

EYELIDS

The eyelids are an extremely sensitive area of the body due to the thinness of skin in this area and ACD is considered the most common dermatologic condition found in association with eyelid dermatitis. The eyelid is a typical site for ectopic contact dermatitis, most commonly caused by allergen from nail varnish or lacquer.[20] Transfer of allergens in hair cosmetics such as p-phenylenediamine (PPD) and ammonium persulfate are widely known to cause a reaction exclusively at the eyelid.[17] Aside from ACD, a differential diagnosis of eyelid dermatitis includes irritant contact dermatitis, protein contact dermatitis, seborrheic dermatitis, atopic eczema, psoriasis, collagen vascular disease, urticaria, rosacea, cutaneous T-cell lymphoma, sarcoidosis, and infections.[21] ACD is presumed to be the most common cause of eyelid dermatitis, occurring in 34% to 74% of patients.[21–23] Patch testing reveals that fragrance components, preservative agents, emulsifiers, hair-care products, and nail cosmetic ingredients such as acrylates are the main cosmetic allergenic agents causing ACD of the eyelids.[24]

Mascara, eyeliner, eye shadow, fake eyelashes, and metal in eyelash curlers are all considered cosmetic sources of eyelid dermatitis.[21,25] Shellac is a commonly used cosmetic agent in mascaras that can cause eyelid dermatitis. In a case report from France, 5 out of 5 patients that were patch tested with shellac had positive reactions.[26] Similarly, a study in the United States found 4 patients referred for evaluation of eyelid dermatitis to have used the same mascara, and shellac was the only individual mascara ingredient to which all 4 patients tested positive.[27]

The NACDG published a study in 2007 that identified a list of 26 top contact allergens that could create a "potential screening series for the evaluation of patients with eyelid dermatitis, without other areas of involvement."[20] Gold tops the list as the most common allergen, accounting for exclusive eyelid dermatitis, and is explained by the release of gold particles in the presence of sweat and abrasive materials, such as titanium dioxide, a common component of facial makeup (an opacifying agent) and sunscreens (blocks ultraviolet light).[28] A patient with metal allergy who wears jewelry may experience this as the gold wears down and the skin is exposed to such substances.

NECK

Similar to the eyelid, the neck is commonly involved in cosmetic-induced ACD due to thinness of the skin and its continual exposure to the environment. ACD affects the neck, either because of products directly applied to the neck or products applied to the face, scalp, and hair that are transferred to the neck, or by contact with metal in jewelry. Nail polish is a well-known cosmetic offender, and a study of ACD from nail varnish determined the face and neck to be the most affected sites. The most common allergen in nail polish was tosylamide formaldehyde resin (TSFR), the ingredient used to create an adhesion between nail polish and the nail.[29] In a separate study, the NACDG found that TSFR was responsible for 4% of positive patch tests.[7] Perfumes are also an obvious source of ACD, as culturally, the neck is the most common place to spray a fragrance. For patients sensitized to fragrances, an "atomizer sign" may develop, wherein repeated application to the neck can cause a focal dermatitis near the prominentia laryngea (Adam's apple).[30] Such a sign may alert a physician to the cause of neck dermatitis and allow early intervention for proper management.

HANDS

Irritant and ACD are the leading causes of hand dermatitis, a common condition that constitutes 20% to 35% of all dermatitis.[31] Aside from irritant and ACD, a differential diagnosis of hand dermatitis includes pompholyx, hyperkeratotic, frictional, nummular, vesicular, and atopic hand dermatitis.[32] ACD of the hands is caused by occupational and nonoccupational allergens, and several studies cite that hairdressing is associated with an increased risk of ACD as compared with the general population.[33–36] A retrospective cross-sectional analysis of positive patch-test reactions focusing on cosmetic allergens found that hairdressing is the most common occupation associated with allergy to cosmetics, and hair products are the most common source of occupation-related reactions.[12] Hands are the most commonly affected site, with rates of hand dermatitis as high as 93% in patch-tested hairdressers and cosmetologists.[37] Studies report an estimated lifetime risk of hand dermatitis in hairdressers and cosmetologists to be 29.1%,[38] 37.6%,[39] and 44.5%.[40]

SCALP

The scalp can be frequently exposed to cosmetic agents, particularly through the use of hair dyes and shampoos. Because of the thickness of skin on the scalp, it is typically uninvolved in ACD unless the patient is particularly sensitive to PPD, a potent sensitizer commonly used in hair dyes. Such sensitization can lead to edema and crusting of the scalp.[17] The Information Network of Departments of Dermatology, a collaborative effort of multiple dermatology departments in Europe that conducts epidemiologic surveillance of contact allergy, patch tested 1320 patients suspected of ACD of the scalp.[41] They found the most common allergens causing adverse reactions to be hair-coloring agents such as PPD, toluene-2,5-diamine, p-aminophenol, 3-aminophenol, and p-aminoazobenzene. A portion of the patients of this study had their own cosmetic products patch tested. Of those items, medical products, hair tints and bleaches, and hair-cleansing products accounted for approximately two-thirds of positive patch-test reactions, with hair tints and bleaches constituting the largest percentage.

Psoriasis, which commonly presents on the scalp, is one particular condition that can be exacerbated by an ACD. Two separate cases reported patients with stable psoriasis that developed pustular psoriatic lesions of the scalp, triggered by an ACD to zinc pyrithione, a component of shampoos that treats dandruff and scalp psoriasis.[42,43] Clinicians should be aware of this potential scalp exacerbation due to ACD.

ANOGENITAL

ACD in the anogenital area is uncommon but a cause of significant discomfort. A retrospective analysis of 1238 patch-tested individuals found only 2.4% of patients with genital dermatitis.[44] It occurs through direct contact with anogenital-specific products such as feminine hygiene products, unintentional contact from nonanogenital products transferred to the area, or through oral administration of substances excreted in urine and feces. Common allergens among patients with anogenital involvement are substances found in products used in the anogenital area (fragrances, preservatives, corticosteroids).[45] Following this, they include fragrance, balsam of Peru, and nickel.[44–46] Spices and flavorings, such as nutmeg, peppermint oil, coriander, curry mix, peppermint oil, and onion powder, are also reported to be associated with anogenital and vulval pruritus and dermatitis.[47,48]

Due to the natural environment of the genital area, the barrier function is frequently compromised by moisture, friction, and heat, rendering it particularly susceptible to ACD.[49] Reactions can be acute or chronic. Acutely, ACD of the vulva can be severely erythematous, edematous, and ulcerative with possible vesicle formation at the site of contact. Chronic ACD of the vulva occurs via extended exposure to a weak allergen, presenting in a pattern of flares and remission characterized by varying degrees of pruritis. Clinically, the vulva appears erythematous or hyperpigmented, marked by lichenified plaques with variable scale and excoriation.[17,50]

COMMON ALLERGENS
Preservatives

Formaldehyde-releasing preservatives: Quaternium-15, Imidazolidinyl urea, Diazolidinyl urea, DMDM hydantoin

Formaldehyde is currently used in a variety of products, such as fertilizers, cleaning products, and waterproof glues; however it is rarely used as a cosmetic preservative because it is a frequent sensitizer.[14] In turn, manufacturers use formaldehyde-releasing preservatives, which include Quaternium-15, Imidazolidinyl urea, Diazolidinyl urea, and DMDM hydantoin,[51] substances that still top the list of allergens causing positive patch-test reactions (**Table 2**). These preservatives are added to numerous skin, hair, and makeup products for their antimicrobial properties. There is legislation in the European Union to limit the amount of these substances in products[52]; in contrast, there is no regulation in the United States on the concentration or use of any formaldehyde-releasing preservatives. According to data from the FDA, approximately 1 in 5 cosmetic products (19.5%) contains a formaldehyde releaser.[53] Cross-reactivity between formaldehyde and formaldehyde-releasers varies, suggesting that allergy to one formaldehyde-releasing preservative does not necessarily restrict the use of the entire class of formaldehyde-releasing preservatives.[51] It is generally understood that the result of a patch test outweighs the theoretical cross-reactions of formaldehyde-releasing preservatives (**Table 3**).

Table 2
Top 10 NACDG standard screening allergens associated with cosmetic source in females and males

Female	Male
Quaternium-15	Quaternium-15
Myroxylon pereirae (balsam of Peru)	Fragrance mix
Fragrance mix	Myroxylon perierae (balsam of Peru)
PPD	Diazolidinyl urea
Methyldibromoglutaronitrile/phenoxyethanol	Imidazolidinyl urea
Formaldehyde	Diazolidinyl urea (not in petrolatum)
TSFR	Cocamidopropyl betaine
Cocamidopropyl betaine	Formaldehyde
Glyceryl thioglycolate	DMDM hydantoin
Diazolidinyl urea	p-Phenylenediamine

Adapted from Warshaw EM, Buchholz HJ, Belsito DV, et al. Allergic patch test reactions associated with cosmetics: retrospective analysis of cross-sectional data from the North American Contact Dermatitis Group, 2001–2004. J Am Acad Dermatol 2009;60(1):30–31; with permission.

Fragrances and Myroxylon Pereirae

Several studies document fragrance mix and *Myroxylon pereirae* (balsam of Peru) as the most common cause of cosmetic ACD,[7,54,55] with 42%–54% of patch-tested patients suspected to have cosmetic dermatitis demonstrating positive reactions.[15,56] Fragrances are ubiquitously used in cosmetic products; aside from its obvious use in colognes and perfumes, they are found in makeup, toothpastes, deodorant, household cleaning products, soaps, medications, and even products that are labeled as "unscented," as they may contain masking fragrance.[57–61]

M pereirae, a naturally produced fragrance from trees of the same name in Central America, contains cinnamic acid, cinnamic aldehyde, methyl cinnamate, benzyl cinnamate, benzyl benzoate, benzoic acid, benzyl alcohol, and vanilla.[62] It is used to screen for fragrance allergy and is reported to detect about 50% of fragrance-sensitive patients.[14,54]

Table 3
Formaldehyde-releasing preservatives

Formaldehyde-releasing Preservative	Special Features
Quaternium-15	• Most common cosmetic preservative allergen • More than 8 times as sensitizing as imidazolidinyl urea • Most common coallergen in patients who react positively to formaldehyde
Imidazolidinyl urea	• Odorless, tasteless, colorless, pH-independent • Previous studies rank this high as a causal cosmetic allergen, but its frequency of causing cosmetic allergy has decreased over time
Diazolidinyl urea	• Structurally related to imidazolidinyl urea, but with wider antimicrobial spectrum • Cross-reacts with imidazolidinyl urea • Sensitization mainly via formaldehyde release, but primary sensitization is possible
DMDM Hydantoin	• Found most frequently in shampoos • Positive patch-test reactions from hair care products highly correlated with DMDM hydantoin
Methyldibromoglutaronitrile (MDBGN)	• Banned in use of all cosmetics and soaps in European Union in 2008; no corresponding US regulation • Increasing rate of MDBGN allergy in Europe and US

Cocamidopropyl Betaine

Cocamidopropyl betaine (CAPB) is a surfactant derived from coconut oil that is used in shampoo, liquid soap, skin cleansers, shower gels, and deodorants.[63,64] CAPB itself is not an allergen. Its allergenic properties are attributed to the impurities involved in its synthesis, dimethylaminopropulamine, and cocamidopropyl dimethylamine (also known as amidoamine or cocamidoamine).[65–67] As of October 2005, 1242 of 22,016 products in the FDA's Voluntary Cosmetic Registration Program contained CAPB.[68]

PPD

This common hair dye ingredient is an oxidizing agent used in permanent or semi-permanent preparations. Recent reports link this potent sensitizer to henna, popularly used in India and the Middle East for temporary tattoos (mehandi) and hair dying.[69,70] It is added to henna to darken the natural shade and can potentially sensitize the patient to develop an ACD if a patient dyes his/her hair later.[71] It is a leading contact allergen in hair products causing eczema of the face and upper trunk in hair-dying customers and a well-known occupation-related cause of allergic hand eczema in hairdressers.[72] Facial dermatitis usually presents proximal to the hairline, but may include the eyelids and neck with possible scalp sparing.[73] Cross-reactivity with other para-amino-group chemicals, such as para-aminobenzoic acid, sulfonamide, procainamide, and hydrochlorothiazide, is possible.[74,75]

Glyceryl Monothioglycolate

Glyceryl monothioglycolate (GMT) is used in acid permanent wave solutions and can persist up to 3 months in the hair.[76] It allows hair to be curled or waved by altering disulfide bonds in hair keratin. An ACD of the scalp caused by GMT can become severe and result in scaling, edema, and crusting.[77] GMT is capable of penetrating rubber gloves, making it a common sensitizer in hairdressers manifesting in reactions on the hands, forearms, face, and neck.[17] It was the second most common allergen in hair products in one study, causing reactions in 17.5% of female patients and 6.7% of male patients.[12]

TSFR

TSFR is the classic cause of ectopic dermatitis due to nail polish. It commonly affects the eyelids, lateral part of the neck, and face; less common areas include the chest and groin.[29,78] It is present in more than 90% of nail polishes in Europe and most lacquers in the United States, forming the product's shiny enamel finish that allows adherence to the nail. Warshaw and colleagues[12] found that 55.6% of 171 female patients with specific allergy to nail products had reactions to TSFR. The allergenic component of TSFR is the resin, not formaldehyde.[79] Nail lacquer can also contain epoxy and (meth)acrylate compounds, and other allergenic copolymers that contribute to a reaction, potentially causing a confusing clinical picture.

Gallates

Propyl gallate, octyl gallate, and dodecyl gallate are all antioxidants used since 1947 to prevent the deterioration of unsaturated fatty acids that can cause product discoloration and odor.[80] Dodecyl gallate has the greatest sensitizing potential according to Hausen and Beyer,[81] but propyl gallate is the most commonly used gallate in the cosmetic industry.[82] It is most often found in waxy or oily lip products, such as lipstick, lip balms, and salves, causing cheilitis.[83,84] Cosmetic creams and lotions may also contain this antioxidant, but infrequently cause ACD because of low concentrations. Cross-reactions between gallates are possible, so a patient that tests positive for one gallate should avoid the entire class of gallates. However, if multiple gallates are tested and the patient does not react to all of them, the patient should only avoid the specific sensitizing gallate.[80]

Patch Testing

The ability of a clinician to obtain a thorough history is crucial for the proper diagnosis and management of a patient with cosmetic allergy. Questions leading to a diagnosis of ACD should include inquiries into skin disease history, use of personal products, occupation, work environment, hobbies and activities, causes of exacerbations and improvements, time since onset, lesion severity, progression, and seasonal variation.

A detailed history should be followed with a careful examination of the lesion. Attention must be paid to the morphology, pattern, and extent of involvement, which can be a clue to the causal cosmetic. Once a diagnosis of ACD is considered, the gold standard to assess ACD properly is the patch test, which will re-expose the patient to suspected allergens under a controlled environment. The answers to the questions from the detailed history and the examination should be used to prepare the proper patches for testing, and the clinician may consider including certain samples of patients' own products.

In 2009, a panel of contact dermatitis experts from the American Contact Dermatitis Society developed an extensive Core Allergen Series intended to be broadly useful for all regions of the United States. Composed of 80 allergens, it is larger than any single series and includes allergens that are present in the existing European Standard Series, the Extended International Series, and the British Contact Dermatitis Series, as well as allergens that are not included in any of those series.[85] A study in 1992 reported that a standard series detects 70% to 80% of all causes of ACD.[86] The series includes some cosmetically relevant allergens such as balsam of Peru, fragrance mix, PPD, colophony, and formaldehyde, but there are many important cosmetic allergens missing. To address this issue, many have studied the value of adding a cosmetic series to the standard series. The findings suggest that adding supplemental allergens to a standard series can increase the diagnostic accuracy of patch testing. By adding 12 supplemental cosmetic allergens, one Swedish study identified 25 of 1075 patch-tested patients who did not react to the standard series, but to the supplemental patches alone.[87] Furthermore, a study conducted in Israel found that 32.8% of patch-tested patients demonstrated a positive reaction to at least one allergen in the cosmetic series.[88] Wetter and colleagues[89] evaluated how useful the addition of a cosmetic series would be to the Mayo Clinic standard series, NACDG standard series, and thin-layer rapid use epicutaneous (TRUE) test. They found that a significant number of patients with skin care product allergy would have been overlooked if the standard series were used alone. The TRUE test alone would have overlooked 22.5% of patients with preservative allergy, 11.3% with fragrance allergy, and 17.3% with vehicle allergy. Results with the NACDG are similar (17.9%, 10.1%, and 17.3%, respectively). A study comparing the European standard series versus supplementation with a cosmetic series found that 15% of patients would have had their allergen sensitivity missed had the standard series been used alone.[90] These findings suggest that in patch testing for cosmetic ACD, it is important to test beyond the baseline series.

The utility of adding a cosmetic series to a standard series depends on the clinical suspicion of a cosmetic contact allergy. Only in the correct and relevant setting will a cosmetic series increase the capability to detect causal allergens, and not all components of the cosmetic series may be necessary. For this reason, a thorough history is important, because it will help doctors to determine the most effective patch test possible for the patient. Moreover, studies have highlighted the importance of including patients' own personal products when considering cosmetic allergy.[12,91]

In the analysis by Warshaw and colleagues, 16.3% of cosmetic-allergic patients reacted solely to a non-NACDG standard allergen; these patients would not have uncovered an offending allergen if tested with the standard series alone. It is important to consider testing a patient's own products.

MANAGEMENT

The cornerstone of management in patients with ACD is avoidance of the triggering allergen. The key to helping a patient do this is to highlight the prevalence of the allergen in various consumer products and to outline the availability of substitutes to achieve successful avoidance. In 1976, the FDA required that ingredients be listed on all consumer cosmetics, which allowed feasibility of allergen avoidance.[92] The United States National Library of Medicine provides a Household Product Database where patients may find information on the specific ingredients found in various cosmetics and household products (hpd.nlm.nih.gov/index. htm).

There are some hurdles to achieve complete ease of management. Fragrances are a ubiquitous and leading cause of contact allergy to cosmetics, but components are not individually listed, because they are considered trade secrets.[92] Similarly, formaldehyde is very commonly used and avoidance can be difficult. One study found that formaldehyde content was incorrectly labeled in 23% to 33% of products they tested.[93]

An invaluable tool for physicians and patients to manage cosmetically induced ACD properly is the Contact Allergen Management Program, managed by the American Contact Dermatitis Society (www. contactderm.org). It is a computerized database of thousands of cosmetics and personal care products that a patient can use to personalize a list of items that are free of the offending allergen. After a patient has been patch tested and the allergen is pinpointed, the offending agent can be entered into the database and a list will be generated of all safe products the patient can use. It makes avoidance of the ingredient causing an allergic reaction more manageable for the patient. Although not an exhaustive list, the database is updated periodically and is a very good resource to manage ACD due to cosmetic use.

Chronic eczematous dermatitis reactions may be encountered when a patient has a chronic sensitivity to a weak allergen. It is more common than acute vesicular eruptions because most cosmetic ingredients are relatively weak allergens. Chronic ACD affecting the hands, feet, and non-flexural areas may be managed with topical corticosteroids. For patients with involvement of the face or intertriginous area, topical calcineurin inhibitors such as tacrolimus 0.1% ointment or pimecrolimus 1% cream may be used.[94]

SUMMARY

As cosmetic products remain ubiquitous, frequently used, and constantly developing, ACD due to cosmetic ingredients is a concern among the general population with a likely higher prevalence than currently thought. Clinicians should be aware of the ways in which patients come into contact with allergens, the clinical presentation of a cosmetic-induced allergic reaction, and common allergens in cosmetic products. Patch testing is the gold standard for diagnosing a delayed type hypersensitivity reaction and may be very useful in ascertaining offending cosmetic allergens, leading to proper and effective management of the patient.

REFERENCES

1. US Food and Drug Administration. The federal food, drug, and cosmetic act subchapter II - definitions. Available at: http://www.fda.gov/RegulatoryInformation/Legislation/FederalFoodDrugandCosmeticActFDCAct/FDCActChaptersIandIIShortTitleandDefinitions/default.htm. Accessed March 15, 2013.
2. Menkart J. An analysis of adverse reactions to cosmetics. Cutis 1979;24(6):599–662.
3. Mehta SS, Reddy BS. Cosmetic dermatitis - current perspectives. Int J Dermatol 2003;42(7):533–42.
4. Engasser PG. Cosmetics and contact dermatitis. Dermatol Clin 1991;9(1):69–80.
5. Eiermann HJ, Larsen W, Maibach HI, et al. Prospective study of cosmetic reactions: 1977-1980. North American Contact Dermatitis Group. J Am Acad Dermatol 1982;6(5):909–17.
6. Romaguera C, Camarasa JM, Alomar A, et al. Patch tests with allergens related to cosmetics. Contact Dermatitis 1983;9(2):167–8.
7. Adams RM, Maibach HI. A five-year study of cosmetic reactions. J Am Acad Dermatol 1985;13(6):1062–9.
8. de Groot AC. Contact allergy to cosmetics: causative ingredients. Contact Dermatitis 1987;17(1):26–34.
9. Nielsen NH, Menne T. Allergic contact sensitization in an unselected Danish population. The Glostrup Allergy Study, Denmark. Acta Derm Venereol 1992;72(6):456–60.
10. Dooms-Goossens A. Cosmetics as causes of allergic contact dermatitis. Cutis 1993;52(5):316–20.
11. Robinson MK, Gerberick GF, Ryan CA, et al. The importance of exposure estimation in the assessment of skin sensitization risk. Contact Dermatitis 2000;42(5):251–9.
12. Warshaw EM, Buchholz HJ, Belsito DV, et al. Allergic patch test reactions associated with cosmetics: retrospective analysis of cross-sectional data from the North American Contact Dermatitis Group, 2001-2004. J Am Acad Dermatol 2009;60(1):23–38.
13. Biebl KA, Warshaw EM. Allergic contact dermatitis to cosmetics. Dermatol Clin 2006;24(2):215–32, vii.
14. Orton DI, Wilkinson JD. Cosmetic allergy: incidence, diagnosis, and management. Am J Clin Dermatol 2004;5(5):327–37.
15. Kohl L, Blondeel A, Song M. Allergic contact dermatitis from cosmetics. Retrospective analysis of 819 patch-tested patients. Dermatology 2002;204(4):334–7.
16. Schnuch A, Szliska C, Uter W. Facial allergic contact dermatitis. Data from the IVDK and review of literature. Hautarzt 2009;60(1):13–21 [in German].
17. Fisher AA, Rietschel R, Fowler JF. Fisher's contact dermatitis. 6th edition. Hamilton (ON): BC Decker; 2008.
18. Soga F, Katoh N, Inoue T, et al. Allergic contact dermatitis as a result of diethyldithiocarbamate in a rubber cosmetic sponge. Contact Dermatitis 2008;58(2):116–7.
19. Helbling I, Beck MH. Rubber sponge applicator responsible for "cosmetic" facial dermatitis. Contact Dermatitis 1998;39(1):43.
20. Rietschel RL, Warshaw EM, Sasseville D, et al. Common contact allergens associated with eyelid dermatitis: data from the North American Contact Dermatitis Group 2003-2004 study period. Dermatitis 2007;18(2):78–81.
21. Guin JD. Eyelid dermatitis: experience in 203 cases. J Am Acad Dermatol 2002;47(5):755–65.
22. Ayala F, Fabbrocini G, Bacchilega R, et al. Eyelid dermatitis: an evaluation of 447 patients. Am J Contact Dermat 2003;14(2):69–74.
23. Temesvari E, Ponyai G, Nemeth I, et al. Periocular dermatitis: a report of 401 patients. J Eur Acad Dermatol Venereol 2009;23(2):124–8.
24. Goossens A. Contact allergic reactions on the eyes and eyelids. Bull Soc Belge Ophtalmol 2004;(292):11–7.
25. Brandrup F. Nickel eyelid dermatitis from an eyelash curler. Contact Dermatitis 1991;25(1):77.
26. Le Coz CJ, Leclere JM, Arnoult E, et al. Allergic contact dermatitis from shellac in mascara. Contact Dermatitis 2002;46(3):149–52.
27. Shaw T, Oostman H, Rainey D, et al. A rare eyelid dermatitis allergen: shellac in a popular mascara. Dermatitis 2009;20(6):341–5.
28. Nedorost S, Wagman A. Positive patch-test reactions to gold: patients' perception of relevance and the role of titanium dioxide in cosmetics. Dermatitis 2005;16(2):67–70 [quiz: 55–66].

29. Lazzarini R, Duarte I, de Farias DC, et al. Frequency and main sites of allergic contact dermatitis caused by nail varnish. Dermatitis 2008;19(6):319–22.

30. Jacob SE, Castanedo-Tardan MP. A diagnostic pearl in allergic contact dermatitis to fragrances: the atomizer sign. Cutis 2008;82(5):317–8.

31. Elston DM, Ahmed DD, Watsky KL, et al. Hand dermatitis. J Am Acad Dermatol 2002;47(2):291–9.

32. Warshaw E, Lee G, Storrs FJ. Hand dermatitis: a review of clinical features, therapeutic options, and long-term outcomes. Am J Contact Dermat 2003;14(3):119–37.

33. Valks R, Conde-Salazar L, Malfeito J, et al. Contact dermatitis in hairdressers, 10 years later: patch-test results in 300 hairdressers (1994 to 2003) and comparison with previous study. Dermatitis 2005;16(1):28–31.

34. Iorizzo M, Parente G, Vincenzi C, et al. Allergic contact dermatitis in hairdressers: frequency and source of sensitisation. Eur J Dermatol 2002;12(2):179–82.

35. Sertoli A, Francalanci S, Acciai MC, et al. Epidemiological survey of contact dermatitis in Italy (1984-1993) by GIRDCA (Gruppo Italiano Ricerca Dermatiti da Contatto e Ambientali). Am J Contact Dermat 1999;10(1):18–30.

36. Bordel-Gomez MT, Miranda-Romero A, Castrodeza-Sanz J. Epidemiology of contact dermatitis: prevalence of sensitization to different allergens and associated factors. Actas Dermosifiliogr 2010;101(1):59–75 [in Spanish].

37. Uter W, Lessmann H, Geier J, et al. Contact allergy to hairdressing allergens in female hairdressers and clients–current data from the IVDK, 2003-2006. J Dtsch Dermatol Ges 2007;5(11):993–1001.

38. Lind ML, Albin M, Brisman J, et al. Incidence of hand eczema in female Swedish hairdressers. Occup Environ Med 2007;64(3):191–5.

39. Lysdal SH, Sosted H, Andersen KE, et al. Hand eczema in hairdressers: a Danish register-based study of the prevalence of hand eczema and its career consequences. Contact Dermatitis 2011;65(3):151–8.

40. Hansen HS, Sosted H. Hand eczema in Copenhagen hairdressers–prevalence and under-reporting to occupational registers. Contact Dermatitis 2009;61(6):361–3.

41. Hillen U, Grabbe S, Uter W. Patch test results in patients with scalp dermatitis: analysis of data of the Information Network of Departments of Dermatology. Contact Dermatitis 2007;56(2):87–93.

42. Jo JH, Jang HS, Ko HC, et al. Pustular psoriasis and the Kobner phenomenon caused by allergic contact dermatitis from zinc pyrithione-containing shampoo. Contact Dermatitis 2005;52(3):142–4.

43. Nielsen NH, Menne T. Allergic contact dermatitis caused by zinc pyrithione associated with pustular psoriasis. Am J Contact Dermat 1997;8(3):170–1.

44. Bhate K, Landeck L, Gonzalez E, et al. Genital contact dermatitis: a retrospective analysis. Dermatitis 2010;21(6):317–20.

45. Warshaw EM, Furda LM, Maibach HI, et al. Anogenital dermatitis in patients referred for patch testing: retrospective analysis of cross-sectional data from the North American Contact Dermatitis Group, 1994-2004. Arch Dermatol 2008;144(6):749–55.

46. Kugler K, Brinkmeier T, Frosch PJ, et al. Anogenital dermatoses–allergic and irritative causative factors. Analysis of IVDK data and review of the literature. J Dtsch Dermatol Ges 2005;3(12):979–86 [in German].

47. Vermaat H, Smienk F, Rustemeyer T, et al. Anogenital allergic contact dermatitis, the role of spices and flavour allergy. Contact Dermatitis 2008;59(4):233–7.

48. Vermaat H, van Meurs T, Rustemeyer T, et al. Vulval allergic contact dermatitis due to peppermint oil in herbal tea. Contact Dermatitis 2008;58(6):364–5.

49. Farage M, Maibach HI. The vulvar epithelium differs from the skin: implications for cutaneous testing to address topical vulvar exposures. Contact Dermatitis 2004;51(4):201–9.

50. Pincus SH. Vulvar dermatoses and pruritus vulvae. Dermatol Clin 1992;10(2):297–308.

51. Herbert C, Rietschel RL. Formaldehyde and formaldehyde releasers: how much avoidance of cross-reacting agents is required? Contact Dermatitis 2004;50(6):371–3.

52. Scientific Committee on Cosmetic Products and Non-food Products. Opinion concerning a clarification on the formaldehyde and para-formaldehyde entry in Directive 76/768/EEC on cosmetic products. 2002. Available at: http://ec.europa.eu/food/fs/sc/sccp/out187_en.pdf. Accessed March 20, 2013.

53. de Groot AC, Veenstra M. Formaldehyde-releasers in cosmetics in the USA and in Europe. Contact Dermatitis 2010;62(4):221–4.

54. de Groot AC, Bruynzeel DP, Bos JD, et al. The allergens in cosmetics. Arch Dermatol 1988;124(10):1525–9.

55. Larsen WG. Perfume dermatitis. J Am Acad Dermatol 1985;12(1 Pt 1):1–9.

56. Malten KE, van Ketel WG, Nater JP, et al. Reactions in selected patients to 22 fragrance materials. Contact Dermatitis 1984;11(1):1–10.

57. Buckley DA, Wakelin SH, Seed PT, et al. The frequency of fragrance allergy in a patch-test population over a 17-year period. Br J Dermatol 2000;142(2):279–83.

58. Heisterberg MV, Menne T, Andersen KE, et al. Deodorants are the leading cause of allergic contact

dermatitis to fragrance ingredients. Contact Dermatitis 2011;64(5):258–64.

59. Johansen JD. Fragrance contact allergy: a clinical review. Am J Clin Dermatol 2003;4(11):789–98.

60. Scheinman PL. Is it really fragrance-free? Am J Contact Dermat 1997;8(4):239–42.

61. Scheinman PL. Exposing covert fragrance chemicals. Am J Contact Dermat 2001;12(4):225–8.

62. Scheinman PL. Allergic contact dermatitis to fragrance: a review. Am J Contact Dermat 1996;7(2):65–76.

63. Fowler JF Jr. Cocamidopropyl betaine: the significance of positive patch test results in twelve patients. Cutis 1993;52(5):281–4.

64. de Groot AC, van der Walle HB, Weyland JW. Contact allergy to cocamidopropyl betaine. Contact Dermatitis 1995;33(6):419–22.

65. Foti C, Bonamonte D, Mascolo G, et al. The role of 3-dimethylaminopropylamine and amidoamine in contact allergy to cocamidopropylbetaine. Contact Dermatitis 2003;48(4):194–8.

66. Moreau L, Sasseville D. Allergic contact dermatitis from cocamidopropyl betaine, cocamidoamine, 3-(dimethylamino)propylamine, and oleamidopropyl dimethylamine: co-reactions or cross-reactions? Dermatitis 2004;15(3):146–9.

67. Fowler JF, Fowler LM, Hunter JE. Allergy to cocamidopropyl betaine may be due to amidoamine: a patch test and product use test study. Contact Dermatitis 1997;37(6):276–81.

68. Jacob SE, Amini S. Cocamidopropyl betaine. Dermatitis 2008;19(3):157–60.

69. Kind F, Scherer K, Bircher AJ. Contact dermatitis to para-phenylenediamine in hair dye following sensitization to black henna tattoos - an ongoing problem. J Dtsch Dermatol Ges 2012;10(8):572–8.

70. Nawaf AM, Joshi A, Nour-Eldin O. Acute allergic contact dermatitis due to para-phenylenediamine after temporary henna painting. J Dermatol 2003;30(11):797–800.

71. Le Coz CJ, Lefebvre C, Keller F, et al. Allergic contact dermatitis caused by skin painting (pseudotattooing) with black henna, a mixture of henna and p-phenylenediamine and its derivatives. Arch Dermatol 2000;136(12):1515–7.

72. Handa S, Mahajan R, De D. Contact dermatitis to hair dye: an update. Indian J Dermatol Venereol Leprol 2012;78(5):583–90.

73. Zapolanski T, Jacob SE. para-Phenylenediamine. Dermatitis 2008;19(3):E20–1.

74. LaBerge L, Pratt M, Fong B, et al. A 10-year review of p-phenylenediamine allergy and related para-amino compounds at the Ottawa Patch Test Clinic. Dermatitis 2011;22(6):332–4.

75. Arroyo MP. Black henna tattoo reaction in a person with sulfonamide and benzocaine drug allergies. J Am Acad Dermatol 2003;48(2):301–2.

76. Morrison LH, Storrs FJ. Persistence of an allergen in hair after glyceryl monothioglycolate-containing permanent wave solutions. J Am Acad Dermatol 1988;19(1 Pt 1):52–9.

77. Parsons LM. Glyceryl monothioglycolate. Dermatitis 2008;19(6):E51–2.

78. Liden C, Berg M, Farm G, et al. Nail varnish allergy with far-reaching consequences. Br J Dermatol 1993;128(1):57–62.

79. Fisher AA. Contact dermatitis. 3rd edition. Philadelphia: Lea & Febiger; 1986.

80. Jacob SE, Caperton CV. Allergen avoidance. Gallates. Dermatitis 2007;18(3). Last two pages of journal. No numbers given.

81. Hausen BM, Beyer W. The sensitizing capacity of the antioxidants propyl, octyl, and dodecyl gallate and some related gallic acid esters. Contact Dermatitis 1992;26(4):253–8.

82. Garcia-Melgares ML, de la Cuadra J, Martin B, et al. Sensitization to gallates: review of 46 cases. Actas Dermosifiliogr 2007;98(10):688–93 [in Spanish].

83. Serra-Baldrich E, Puig LL, Gimenez Arnau A, et al. Lipstick allergic contact dermatitis from gallates. Contact Dermatitis 1995;32(6):359–60.

84. Athavale NV, Srinivas CR. Contact cheilitis from propyl gallate in lipstick. Contact Dermatitis 1994;30(5):307.

85. Lee J, Warshaw E, Zirwas MJ. Allergens in the American Contact Dermatitis Society Core Series. Clin Dermatol 2011;29(3):266–72.

86. James WD, Rosenthal LE, Brancaccio RR, et al. American Academy of Dermatology Patch Testing Survey: use and effectiveness of this procedure. J Am Acad Dermatol 1992;26(6):991–4.

87. Lindberg M, Tammela M, Bostrom A, et al. Are adverse skin reactions to cosmetics underestimated in the clinical assessment of contact dermatitis? A prospective study among 1075 patients attending Swedish patch test clinics. Acta Derm Venereol 2004;84(4):291–5.

88. Trattner A, Farchi Y, David M. Cosmetics patch tests: first report from Israel. Contact Dermatitis 2002;47(3):180–1.

89. Wetter DA, Yiannias JA, Prakash AV, et al. Results of patch testing to personal care product allergens in a standard series and a supplemental cosmetic series: an analysis of 945 patients from the Mayo Clinic Contact Dermatitis Group, 2000-2007. J Am Acad Dermatol 2010;63(5):789–98.

90. Ada S, Seckin D. Patch testing in allergic contact dermatitis: is it useful to perform the cosmetic series in addition to the European standard series? J Eur Acad Dermatol Venereol 2010;24(10):1192–6.

91. Uter W, Balzer C, Geier J, et al. Patch testing with patients' own cosmetics and toiletries–results of the IVDK*, 1998-2002. Contact Dermatitis 2005; 53(4):226–33.

92. Greif M, Maibach HI. United States cosmetic ingredient labeling. Contact Dermatitis 1977; 3(2):94–7.

93. Rastogi SC. Analytical control of preservative labelling on skin creams. Contact Dermatitis 2000;43(6): 339–43.

94. Belsito D, Wilson DC, Warshaw E, et al. A prospective randomized clinical trial of 0.1% tacrolimus ointment in a model of chronic allergic contact dermatitis. J Am Acad Dermatol 2006;55(1):40–6.

Next Generation Cosmeceuticals
The Latest in Peptides, Growth Factors, Cytokines, and Stem Cells

Sarah Malerich, BS[a],*, Diane Berson, MD[b]

KEYWORDS

• Cosmeceuticals • Stem cells • Growth factors • Peptides • Photoaging • Rhytides • Cytokines

KEY POINTS

• Collagen, elastin, and other components of the skin diminish with age and may be replaced through the use of cosmeceuticals.
• Peptides induce neocollagenesis replacing lost extracellular matrix and reducing the appearance of wrinkles.
• Cosmeceuticals containing growth factors and cytokines involved in wound repair aid in the repair of chronic damage to the skin.
• Allogenic stem cells derived from human adipocytes produce growth factors which promote fibroblasts within the skin along with promoting wound healing.
• Xenogenic stem cells derived from plants have anti-senescent properties.

INTRODUCTION

As the population grows, there is a particular increase in the middle-aged and elderly population, the so-called "baby boomers." Among this population is a continued increase in the desire for younger looking skin. Areas of particular concern include loss of elasticity, rhytides, irregular texture, pigmentation, and dryness.[1,2] This desire has led to the development of cosmeceuticals, which are in between cosmetics and physiologically altering pharmaceuticals.

Aging occurs by two mechanisms: intrinsic and extrinsic aging. Intrinsic aging is inevitable and results in atrophy, fibroblast reduction, and thinning blood vessels.[3] Collagen is particularly affected, as the synthesis steadily declines with age.[4]

Likewise, elastin also declines with age.[4,5] Extrinsic aging primarily results from the effects of UV damage. Other causes include environmental factors, such as smoking, pollution, and poor nutrition.[3,6] This type of damage leads to increased degradation of collagen and elastin. Aged skin shows a decrease in extracellular matrix (ECM) proteins, increased collagen degradation, and decreased fibroblasts.[7] Furthermore, there is a reduction in the immune response, wound repair, and fiber synthesis.[8] Extrinsic aging leads to the production of free radicals, which in turn activate matrix metalloproteinases (MMPs). This activation of MMPs also leads to ECM degradation.[9] Additionally, free radicals inhibit the tissue inhibitors of metalloproteinase (TIMPs). The goal of

Disclosures: Dr D. Berson is a consultant for Proctor and Gamble, Allergan, Galderma, Rock Creek Pharmaceuticals, La Roche Posay, and Anacor.
[a] Lake Erie College of Osteopathic Medicine, 5000 Lakewood Ranch Boulevard, Bradenton, FL 34211, USA;
[b] Weill Medical College, Cornell University, New York-Presbyterian, 211 East 53rd Street, Suite 3, New York, NY 10022, USA
* Corresponding author.
E-mail address: Sarah.Malerich@med.lecom.edu

Dermatol Clin 32 (2014) 13–21
http://dx.doi.org/10.1016/j.det.2013.09.003
0733-8635/14/$ – see front matter © 2014 Elsevier Inc. All rights reserved.

cosmeceuticals is to mitigate some of these effects of aging.

Effective cosmeceuticals must be able to penetrate through the stratum corneum while maintaining their effectiveness. They also must have visible benefits without impacting the skin's barrier function.[10] There has been a recent surge of new cosmeceuticals, and this article discusses the functions, limits, and benefits of peptides, growth factors, cytokines, and stem cells used in these products.

PEPTIDES

Peptides are short amino acid chains with a functional ability to alter skin physiology.[11] The basic cosmetic mechanism behind peptides is to increase collagen production, replacing lost ECM and reducing the size and appearance of wrinkles. Peptides are able to regulate fibroblast production of ECM components,[12,13] mainly through the use of signal peptides. It is hypothesized that the introduction of subfragments of these components, such as elastin and collagen, will act as feedback stimulators inducing their own synthesis.[11]

Use of peptides for topical application is limited by the ionic nature of the amino acid chains.[14] However, this may be circumvented through the incorporation of a lipophilic derivative, such as palmitoyl. Peptides generally have a short half-life when delivered orally because of significant first-pass effect. By delivering them transdermally, fully functional peptides may be delivered to the desired site. The length and membrane permeability are important when assessing them for use in cosmeceuticals.[15] Addition of peptides to products can get very costly; however, minimal compositions of peptides have shown significant results. Peptides are thus very potent and require only minor amounts, minimizing cost.

Signal Peptides

This discussion focuses on signal peptides, which stimulate ECM production, specifically increasing collagen synthesis. A list of functional peptides found in cosmeceuticals can be found in **Table 1**. One of the longest used peptides, oligopeptide-20, consists of 12 amino acids. This peptide increases collagen and hyaluronic acid in cultured keratinocytes and fibroblasts.[16] Another peptide shown to increase collagen production is palmitoyl pentapeptide-4 (Pal KTTKS). Pal KTTKS is a fragment of procollagen I. It increases production of collagen I and III through the stimulation of fibroblasts, and also stimulates production of fibronectin and elastin.[10,17,18] The palmitoyl derivative was added to the pentapeptide, increasing its lipophilic properties and enhancing absorption. Pal

KTTKS also inhibited the production of glycoasaminoglycans in the skin, an increase of which is associated with increased age and photodamaged skin.[19]

Palmitoyl-lysine-threonine (pal-KT) is one of the shortest peptides. When tested with human skin equivalents, it was found to enhance differentiation of the epidermis, basement membrane zone, and dermal fibroblasts.[20] Within dermal fibroblasts, pal-KT increased collagen I, collagen IV, and fibronectin.

The hexapeptide, consisting of amino acids val-gly-val-ala-pro-gly, is an elastin fragment with chemotactic properties. It attracts cells to wound sites[10] and significantly stimulates fibroblast proliferation within human skin.[11] It also decreases the expression of elastin.[21] Conversely, this peptide has been found in another study[3] to induce proteolytic and inflammatory damage by upregulation of MMP-1 and MMP-3, requiring further study.

Tripeptide-10 citrulline (T10-C) is a decorin-like molecule. Decorin is a leucine-rich proteoglycan directly involved in matrix organization. By binding to the surface of collagen molecules, decorin regulates their interaction with other collagen molecules, stabilizing and orienting them, thus establishing a uniform tissue shape. This mechanism increases the tensile strength of collagen and reduces collagen disruption. With age, however, comes a lack of functional decorin within the skin.[22] Instead, it is replaced with a truncated, nonfunctional fragment known as decorunt.

T10-C contains the collagen-binding site sequences of decorin and, like decorin, is able to regulate collagen fibers. Unlike other peptides, which increase the quantity of collagen, it increases the quality of the collagen, enhancing uniformity and increasing cohesion. T10-C showed a decrease in collagen fiber diameter, similar to decorin, which led to increased skin suppleness and firmness.[23] Another peptide, arg-gly-asp-ser, enhances ECM structure. This tetrapeptide is a fragment of fibronectin and enhances cell and collagen cohesiveness.[10]

Peptamide-6 is derived from the yeast *Saccharomyces*. It is a firming peptide that works by upregulation of growth factors and increasing collagen synthesis. This peptide has been shown to improve skin elasticity and deformation response.[23]

Acetyl tetrapepide-9 and -11 (AcTP1 and AcTP2, respectively) increase skin thickness and firmness. AcTP1 increases collagen I and lumican synthesis. AcTP2 stimulates keratinocyte growth and syndecan-1 synthesis.[24]

In addition to their effects on the ECM, peptides may also function as skin whitening agents. PKEK,

Table 1
Peptides used as cosmeceutical ingredients

Antiaging Effect	Peptide Type	Peptide	Mechanism
Wrinkle and fine line reduction	Signal	Arg-gly-asp-ser	Increases cell-cell cohesion
		Oligopeptide-20	Increases collagen and hyaluronic acid
		Pal-KTTKS	Increases collagen I and III, fibronectin, and elastin
			Inhibits glycoasaminoglycans formation
		Pal-KT	Induces differentiation of the epidermis, BM zone, and fibroblasts
			Increases collagen I, collagen IV, and fibronectin
		Amino acids val-gly-val-ala-pro-gly	Stimulates fibroblast proliferation
	Carrier and signal	Glycyl-L-histidyl-L-lysine	Enhances collagen production
			Cu complex inhibits TIMP-1 and -2, increases levels of MMP-1 and -2, and increases synthesis of dermatan sulfate and heparin sulfate
	Enzyme inhibiting	Tyr-tyr-arg-ala-asp-asp-ala	Inhibits procollagen C proteinase
Wrinkle improvement, firming	Signal	AcTP1	Increases collagen I and lumican synthesis
		AcTP2	Stimulates keratinocyte growth and syndecan-1 synthesis
		T10-C	Mimics decorin
			Increases collagen fiber uniformity and enhances cohesion
Skin firming	Signal	Peptamide-6	Increases collagen synthesis
			Upregulates growth factors
Skin whitening	Signal	PKEK	Reduces IL-6, IL-8, tumor necrosis factor-α, proopiomelanocorticotropin, α-melanocyte-stimulating hormone, tyrosinase

Abbreviations: AcTP1, acetyl tetrapepide-9; AcTP2, acetyl tetrapepide-11; Pal-KT, palmitoyl-lysine-threonine; Pal-KTTKS, palmitoyl pentapeptide-4; T10-C, tripeptide-10 citrulline.

a tetrapeptide of amino acids pro-lys-glu-lys, reduces pigmentation by reducing the expression of interleukin (IL) -6, IL-8, tumor necrosis factor-α, proopiomelanocorticotropin, α-melanocyte-stimulating hormone, and tyrosinase secondary to UVB upregulation of these genes.[25] Skin pigmentation is thus decreased by reduction of UVB-induced proinflammatory reactions.

Sirtuin genes may also be altered through the application of peptides. A biopeptide developed from the yeast *Kluyveromyces* has been shown to stimulate sirtuins within human skin cells,[26] specifically SIRT1. Sirtuins enhance cell longevity by allowing transcription to occur. This occurs through deacetylation of silenced genes. SIRT1

has also been shown to increase manganese superoxide dismutase, resulting in enhanced repair of oxidative stress.[27] Sirtuins are decreased in aging skin and it can thus be hypothesized that increasing them will result in skin longevity. Topical application reduces wrinkles and pigmented spots, along with improving skin texture and hydration.[26]

Enzyme-Inhibiting Peptides

Another type of peptide is the enzyme-inhibiting peptide. One of these is made up of the amino acid chain tyr-tyr-arg-ala-asp-asp-ala. This inhibits procollagen C proteinase, whose function is to cleave a portion of type I procollagen. By inhibiting this enzyme, there is a reduced destruction of procollagen.[28]

Carrier Peptides

Carrier peptides are another subtype. Peptides, such as glycyl-L-histidyl-L-lysine, have been shown to facilitate copper uptake by cells.[29] Copper has beneficial effects on the skin and is required for wound healing.[11] Alone, this tripeptide also enhances collagen production.[11] Together, the Cu-tripeptide complex facilitates dermal remodeling through inhibition of TIMPs 1 and 2, and increasing levels of MMP-1 and -2.[30] Specifically within fibroblasts, this complex increases synthesis of dermatan sulfate and heparin sulfate.[31]

Potency and Adverse Effects

Among the peptides discussed, effects are generally seen in about 8 weeks with twice daily application. Mixtures between 3 and 10 ppm exhibit efficacy, indicating high potency. PKEK required the most active ingredient, 40 ppm, to generate the desired effect. No significant adverse effects were seen, including redness, burning, or itching. Likewise, there was no impact on skin barrier function, based on transepidermal water loss measurements. Improvements were seen in wrinkles, fine lines, and skin roughness.

GROWTH FACTORS AND CYTOKINES

Many growth factors are involved in wound healing, both chronic and acute. Growth factors have been introduced into the cosmeceutical world based on the hypothesis that the aging process of skin is similar to that of a chronic wound.[9] Their ability to increase fibroblast and keratinocyte proliferation within the dermis, thus inducing ECM formation, supports this idea.[7] Aging skin has reduced amounts of fibroblasts and decreased levels of growth factors. By supplementing these normal growth factors, we may allow for the natural repair of skin.

Growth factors are produced and secreted by many cell types of the skin, including fibroblasts, keratinocytes, and melanocytes. Included within these secreted growth factors are those that regulate the immune system, also known as cytokines. Cytokines are also involved in skin repair.[32] Many growth factors are involved in wound repair and thus most of the topical products contain a combination of growth factors. It is important to combine growth factors and cytokines because they work together and regulate each other throughout the healing process. A general overview of the growth factors and cytokines found in cosmetic products and their functions can be found in **Table 2**.

One of the concerns with growth factors, as with other peptides, is their size and ability to penetrate the epidermis. Growth factors and cytokines are very large molecules, usually more than 15,000 Da, and are hydrophilic.[33] However, it is proposed that absorption occurs by way of hair follicles, sweat glands, and compromised skin.[34–36] Once absorbed into the epidermis, communication is able to occur between epidermal cells and cells of the dermal layers.[37,38] Growth factors are also very unstable outside of their physiologically active environment unless stored at $-20°C$, which is clearly not practical for the use of cosmetic application. One study,[39] however, showed that growth factors and cytokines remained stable for more than 24 months.

Growth factors regulate cell growth and thus have a potential for carcinogenic transformation of cells.[9] This is proposed to be largely based on the presence of vascular endothelial growth factor (VEGF). Receptors for VEGF are present on some types of melanoma cells.[40] However, increased VEGF in melanoma has had conflicting results. One study has shown an increase in melanoma cell proliferation when cells were combined with VEGF, whereas another failed to do so.[41,42] A Food and Drug Administration investigation of a growth factor product determined that very large concentrations of growth factors, much higher than the levels found in topical cosmeceutical products, are required for this potential.[9] Furthermore, because of the large size, minimal amounts of growth factors enter the skin. Thus, topical application of growth factors is unlikely to have any effect on cancer growth.[40]

Topical transforming growth factor (TGF)-β1 has been shown to restore damaged skin and increase epidermal thickening and the Grenz zone layer; histologic studies have shown increased epidermal thickness and fibroblast density.[43] A reduction of solar elastosis was also seen, particularly among patients with more severe photodamage. An increased number of smaller-diameter collagen fibers were seen demonstrating neocollagenesis. There was a decrease in the appearance of wrinkles.[44] Patients reported improved skin elasticity, texture, hydration, lines, and wrinkles, along with decreased skin tightness.[43]

One source for growth factors, cytokines, and matrix proteins is neonatal dermal fibroblasts, which secrete more than 110 of these combined products.[33,45] A study of applications of these

Table 2
Growth factors and cytokines found in cosmeceutical products

Growth factors	Fibroblast growth factor	Activates fibroblasts, angiogenic, induces collagen synthesis
	Heparin binding-epidermal growth factor	Keratinocyte and fibroblast mitogen
	Hepatocyte growth factor	Tissue regeneration and wound healing
	Insulin-like growth factor	Activates fibroblasts and endothelial cells
	Placenta growth factor	Activates fibroblasts, promotes endothelial growth
	Platelet-derived growth factor	Induces fibroblast migration, fibroblast mitogen, matrix production
	Transforming growth factor-β1	Induces keratinocyte, fibroblast, and macrophage migration, and angiogenesis Initiates collagen and fibronectin synthesis; modulates degradation of matrix proteins
	Transforming growth factor-β2	Induces keratinocyte, fibroblast, and macrophage migration; initiates collagen and fibronectin synthesis
	Transforming growth factor-β3	Antiscarring
	Vascular endothelial growth factor	Inhibits collagen and hyaluronic acid degradation
Cytokines	IL-1α and -1β	Activates growth factor expression in macrophages, keratinocytes, and fibroblasts
	IL-1ra	Anti-inflammatory
	IL-10	Anti-inflammatory
	IL-13	Anti-inflammatory
	Tumor necrosis factor-α	Activates growth factor expression in macrophages, keratinocytes, and fibroblasts

products shows a statistically significant decrease in wrinkles and fine lines along with an increase in Grenz zone collagen and epidermal thickness after topical application to Fitzpatrick skin types II and higher.[46] These effects were found to last at least 3 months after the discontinuation of treatment. Improvements were also shown in skin roughness and shadows after topical application to mild to severe photodamaged skin. This was particularly evident among those with more severe photodamage.[45]

Processed skin-cell proteins from cultured fetal dermal fibroblasts contain a mixture of more than 100 growth factors and cytokines (**Box 1**).[3] Fetal fibroblasts have been used for wound healing in the pediatric population and have been shown to produce complete closure.[47] Experiments have shown that a decrease in TGF-β1 and TGF-β2, and an increase in TGF-β3 are associated with the scarless repair seen in fetal skin.[3,48]

Potency and Adverse Effects

After 2 months of twice daily application, improvements of wrinkles in the periorbital and perioral

areas were seen. Reduced dark under-eye color was noted, and improved texture and firmness. These effects may have resulted from increased collagen production of the skin under the eyes. Thicker skin aids in the ability to cover the underlying vessels responsible for the appearance of dark circles.[49] Improvements became statistically significant after 30 days of treatment and continued to improve for the remainder of the 6 weeks. Cheek skin was also noted to be tighter and firmer.

Growth factors are safe and have not been associated with any risks, although there is a potential for allergic reaction in hypersensitive patients.[40] Topical application produces increased collagen generation, thickening of the epidermis, and improvements in skin texture and wrinkles.[46]

STEM CELLS

Stem cells are being studied for their potential use in cosmetics. These products, which include serums and creams, can contain many stem cell extracts to renew, generate, and repair skin. A stem cell is one that can divide and proliferate, constantly renewing itself, and can subsequently

> **Box 1**
> **Growth factors and cytokines found within processed skin-cell proteins from cultured fetal dermal fibroblasts**
>
> - Beta-nerve growth factor
> - Epidermal growth factor
> - Fibroblast growth factor-2, -4, -6, -7, -9
> - Granulocyte colony–stimulating factor
> - Granulocyte-macrophage colony–stimulating factor
> - Hepatocyte growth factor
> - Insulin-like growth factor-1
> - IL-1α
> - IL-1β
> - IL-1ra (IL-1 receptor antagonist)
> - IL-6
> - IL-8
> - IL-10
> - IL-12
> - IL-13
> - Interferon-γ
> - Platelet-derived growth factor
> - Placenta growth factor
> - TGF-β1
> - TGF-β3
> - TIMP-1
> - TIMP-2
> - Tumor necrosis factor-α
> - VEGF

> **Box 2**
> **Components of ASC-CM**
>
> - Fibroblast growth factor
> - Fibronectin
> - Hepatocyte growth factor
> - Insulin-like growth factor–binding protein 1 and 2
> - Keratinocyte growth factor
> - Macrophage colony–stimulating factor receptor
> - Placenta growth factor
> - Platelet-derived growth factor-AA, and receptor -β
> - Transforming growth factor-β1, -β2
> - Type 1 collagen
> - Vascular endothelial growth factor

be differentiated. Stem cells can be used in cosmeceutical products; they are extracted from animal or plant sources and then cultured in the laboratory to yield extracts of the stem cells. Sources include human adipose tissue; sheep and cow placentas; and plant sources, such as Swiss apple seed.

Allogenic stem cells for dermatologic use arise from human adipocytes. Adipose tissue is abundant in mesenchymal stem cells (MSC), which show an ability to regenerate damaged skin.[50–52] Conditioned media of adipose-derived stem cells (ASC-CM), which are stable, have potential benefits when applied topically. Growth factors produced in ASCs can promote collagen synthesis by dermal fibroblasts.[53,54] Growth factors and other components found to be upregulated within the cultured medium can be found in **Box 2**.[55,56] Furthermore, ASCs promote wound healing,

improve wrinkling, and inhibit melanogenesis.[57–60] They can be used to replace lost soft tissue through the induction of ASCs into adipocytes.[61]

ASCs are similar to other MSCs, including bone marrow–derived stem cells,[50] with respect to cell-surface receptor exhibition, morphology, and their differentiation capacity.[62,63] Surface markers expressed by ASCs and MSCs include those for adhesion molecules, cell surface enzymes, ECM proteins, and glycoproteins.[64–66] They also both secrete collagen, fibronectin, VEGF, hepatocyte growth factor, and fibroblast growth factor.[53,67,68] Cluster of differentiation 90, a marker for MSCs, was found on more than 80% of ASCs.[58]

ASCs stimulate collagen synthesis and decrease MMP-1 levels. They also stimulate the migration of dermal fibroblasts resulting in wrinkle improvements, and protect fibroblasts from oxidative stress induced by UVB irradiation.[50,59] ASC-CM significantly enhanced glutathione peroxidase activity resulting in part of this antioxidative function.[59] They also are able to lighten skin through inhibition of melanin synthesis and tyrosinase activity in a dose-dependent manner.[58] Anti-inflammatory properties result from the secretion of ILs, hepatocyte growth factor, and TGF-β1, which modulate lymphocytic activities.[50] It was shown that caspase-3 activity induced by t-butyl hydroperoxide treatment was reversed by pretreatment with ASC-CM,[59] thus promoting its antiapoptotic capabilities.[57,59,60]

Whitening effects of ASC-CM results from the downregulation of tyrosinase and tyrosinase-related protein 1. These effects have been shown to be mediated by TGF-β1, because reversal of these effects was observed after knock-out of TGF-β1. It has been shown that this reduction of tyrosinase and tyrosinase-related protein 1 is not caused by the inhibition of mRNA expression, but rather by an increased rate of degradation of these molecules.[58]

Stem cells derived from plants include the Uttwiler Spatlauber apple tree from Switzerland and jasmine and lilac seeds.[69] This particular apple tree was chosen because of its prolonged storage properties. The hypothesis is that they prolong longevity when mixed with a person's endogenous stem cells. These cells have been shown to reverse or delay senescence, the natural process of aging. Fibroblasts were incubated with 2% stem cell extract after induction of senescence using H_2O_2 treatment.[69] This was identified by an upregulation or neutralization in several genes important for cellular growth and proliferation. Likewise, isolated hair follicles maintained in growth medium were also shown to have a slightly prolonged growth phase, by 4 days.[69]

Potency and Adverse Effects

Clinically, products containing 2% Uttwiler Spatlauber stem cell extract have been shown to significantly reduce wrinkles in as little as 2 weeks.[56,69–71] However, studies are required to determine the exact mechanisms behind these results and the duration of effectiveness. Although still lacking rigorous data of extensive human studies and research on stem cells, interest continues to rise.

SUMMARY

Cosmeceuticals are a safe and effective way to improve the undesired effects of aging. There are various agents that can be applied to address wrinkles, fine lines, and hyperpigmentation. Cosmeceuticals exert local effects, without systemic absorption. They are also generally well tolerated and no major adverse effects have been observed. Many different options exist, including peptides, growth factors, cytokines, and stem cells, which have joined the cosmeceutical armamentarium.

REFERENCES

1. Griffiths CE, Russman AN, Majmudar G, et al. Restoration of collagen formation in photodamaged human skin by tretinoin (retinoic acid). N Engl J Med 1993;329:530–5.
2. Wlaschek M, Tantcheva-Poor I, Naderi L, et al. Solar UV irradiation and dermal photoaging. J Photochem Photobiol B 2001;63:41–51.
3. Rangarajan V, Dreher F. Topical growth factors for skin rejuvenation. In: Farage MA, Miller KW, Mailbach HI, editors. Textbook of aging skin. Berlin: Springer-Verlag; 2010. p. 1079–87.
4. Uitto J. The role of elastin and collagen in cutaneous aging: intrinsic aging versus photoexposure. J Drugs Dermatol 2008;7(Suppl 2):s12–6.
5. Seite S, Zucchi H, Septier D, et al. Elastin changes during chronological and photo-aging: the important role of lysozyme. J Eur Acad Dermatol Venereol 2006;20:980–7.
6. Baumann L. Skin ageing and its treatment. J Pathol 2007;211:241–51.
7. Gold MH, Goldman MP, Biron J. Efficacy of novel skin cream containing mixture of human growth factors and cytokines for skin rejuvenation. J Drugs Dermatol 2007;6(2):197–201.
8. Sauder DN. Effect of age on epidermal immune function. Dermatol Clin 1986;4:447–54.
9. Sundaram H, Mehta R, Norine JA, et al. Topically applied phsyiologically balanced growth factors: a new paradigm of skin rejuvenation. J Drugs Dermatol 2009;8(5):4–13.
10. Lintner K. Promoting production in the extracellular matrix without compromising barrier. Cutis 2002; 70S:13–6.
11. Lupo MP. Cosmeceutical peptides. Dermatol Surg 2005;31:832–6.
12. Langholz O, Rockel D, Mauch C, et al. Collagen and collagenase gene expression in three dimensional collagen lattices are differently regulated by alpha I beta I and alpha II beta I integrins. J Cell Biol 1995;131(6 Pt 2):1903–15.
13. Katayama K, Seger JM, Raghow R, et al. Regulation of extracellular matrix production by chemically synthesized subfragments of type I collagen carboxy propeptide. Biochemistry 1991;30:7097–104.
14. Robinson LR, Fitzgerald NC, Doughty DG, et al. Topical palmitoyl pentapeptide provides improvement in photoaged human facial skin. Int J Cosmet Sci 2005;27(3):155–60.
15. Blanes-Mira C, Clemente J, Jodas G, et al. A synthetic hexapeptide (Argireline) with anti-wrinkle activity. Int J Cosmet Sci 2002;24:303–10.
16. Varvaresou A, Papageorgiou S, Protopapa E, et al. Efficacy and tolerance study of an oligopeptide with potential anti-aging activity. J Chem Dermatol Sci Appl 2011;1:133–40.
17. Katayama K, Armendariz-Borunda J, Raghow R, et al. A pentapeptide from type I procollagen promotes extracellular matrix production. J Biol Chem 1993;268(14):9941–4.
18. Lintner K. Promoting ECM production without compromising barrier. Cutis 2002;129:S105.
19. Gonzalez S, Moran M, Kochevar I. Chronic photodamage in skin of mast cell-deficient mice. Photochem Photobiol 1999;70:248–53.

20. Osborne R, Mullins LA, Jarrold BB, et al. In vitro skin structure benefits with a new anti-aging peptide, Pal-KT. J Am Acad Dermatol 2008;58(2):AB25.

21. Tajima S, Wachi H, Uemura Y, et al. Modulation by elastin peptide VGVAPG of cell proliferation and elastin expression in human skin fibroblasts. Arch Dermatol Res 1997;289(8):489–92.

22. Puig A, Garcia Anton JM, Mangues M. A new decorin-like tetrapeptide for optimal organization of collagen fibres. Int J Cosmet Sci 2008;30:97–104.

23. Gorouhi F, Maibach HI. Role of topical peptides in preventing or treating aged skin. Int J Cosmet Sci 2009;31:327–45.

24. Pauly G, Contet-Audonneau J, Moussou P, et al. Small proteoglycans in the skin: new targets in the fight against aging. Int J Cosmet Sci 2009; 31(2):154.

25. Marini A, Farwick M, Grether-Beck S, et al. Modulation of skin pigmentation by the tetrapeptide PKEK: in vitro and in vivo evidence for skin whitening effects. Exp Dermatol 2011;21:140–6.

26. Moreau M, Neveu M, Stephan S, et al. Enhancing cell longevitiy for cosmetic application: a complementary approach. J Drugs Dermatol 2007;6:s14–9.

27. Giannaku ME, Partridge L. The interaction between FOXO and SIRT-1: tipping the balance towards survival. Trends Cell Biol 2004;14:408–12.

28. Njieha FK, Morikava T, Tuderman L, et al. Partial purifications of a procollagen C-proteinase. Inhibition by synthetic peptides and sequential cleavage of type I procollagen. Biochemistry 1982;21:757–64.

29. Pickart L, Freedman JH, Loher WJ, et al. Growth-modulating plasma tripeptide may function by facilitating copper uptake into cells. Nature 1980; 288:715–7.

30. Simeon A, Emonard H, Hornebeck W, et al. The tripeptide-copper complex glycyl-L-histidyl-L-lysine-Cu^{2+} stimulates matrix metalloproteinase-2 expression by fibroblast cultures. Life Sci 2000; 67:2257–65.

31. Wegrowski Y, Maquart FX, Borel JP. Stimulation of sulfated glycosaminoglycan synthesis by the tripeptide-copper complex glycyl-L-histidyl-L-lysin-Cu^{2+}. Life Sci 1992;51:1049–56.

32. Eming SA, Krieg T, Davidson JM. Inflammation in wound repair: molecular and cellular mechanisms. J Invest Dermatol 2007;127(3):514–25.

33. Mehta RC, Fitzpatrick RE. Endogenous growth factors as cosmeceuticals. Dermatol Ther 2007;20(5): 350–9.

34. Lademann J, Otbert N, Jacobi U, et al. Follicular penetration and targeting. J Investig Dermatol Symp Proc 2005;10:301–3.

35. Jakasa I, Verberk MM, Bunge AL, et al. Increased permeability for polyethylene glycols through skin compromised by sodium lauryl sulphate. Exp Dermatol 2006;15:801–7.

36. Schaefer H, Lademann J. The role of follicular penetration. A differential view. Skin Pharmacol Appl Skin Physiol 2001;17(Suppl I):23–7.

37. Werner S, Krieg T, Smola H. Keratinocyte-fibroblast interaction in wound healing. J Invest Dermatol 2007;127:998–1008.

38. Ansel J, Perry P, Brown J, et al. Cytokine modulation of keratinocyte cytokines. J Invest Dermatol 1990;94(Suppl 6):s101–7.

39. Banga AK. Transdermal and topical delivery of therapeutic peptides and proteins. In: Therapeutic peptides and proteins: formulation, processing, and delivery systems. 2nd edition. Boca Raton (FL): CRC Press; 2005. p. 259–81.

40. Fitzpatrick RE. Endogenous growth factors as cosmeceuticals. Dermatol Surg 2005;31:827–31.

41. Liu B, Earl HM, Baban D, et al. Melanoma cell lines express VEGF receptor KDR and respond to exogenously added VEGF. Biochem Biophys Res Commun 1995;217:721–7.

42. Graeven U, Fiedler W, Karpinski S, et al. Melanoma-associated expression of vascular endothelial growth factor and its receptor FLT-1 and KDR. J Cancer Res Clin Oncol 1999;125: 621–9.

43. Hussain M, Phelps R, Goldberg DJ. Clinical, histologic, and ultrastructural changes after use of human growth factor and cytokine skin cream for the treatment of skin rejuvenation. J Cosmet Laser Ther 2008;10:104–9.

44. Fisher GJ, Kang S, Varani J, et al. Mechanisms of photoaging and chronological skin aging. Arch Dermatol 2002;138:1462–70.

45. Mehta RC, Smith SR, Grove GL, et al. Reduction in facial photodamage by a topical growth factor product. J Drugs Dermatol 2008;7:864–71.

46. Fitzpatrick RE, Rostan EF. Reversal of photodamage with topical growth factors: a pilot study. J Cosmet Laser Ther 2003;5(1):25–34.

47. Hohlfeld J, de Buys Roessingh A, Hirt-Burri N, et al. Tissue engineered fetal skin constructs for pediatric burns. Lancet 2005;366:484–9.

48. Cass DL, Meuli M, Adzick NS. Scar wars: implications of fetal wound healing for the pediatric burn patient. Pediatr Surg Int 1997;12:484–9.

49. Lupo ML, Cohen JL, Rendon MI. Novel eye cream containing a mixture of human growth factors and cytokines for periorbital skin rejuvenation. J Drugs Dermatol 2007;6(7):725–9.

50. Yang J, Hyung-Min C, Chong-Hyun W, et al. Potential application of adipose-derived stem cells and their secretory factors to skin: discussion from both clinical and industrial viewpoints. Expert Opin Biol Ther 2010;10(4):495–503.

51. Zuk PA, Zhu M, Ashjian P, et al. Human adipose tissue is a source of multipotent stem cells. Mol Biol Cell 2002;13(12):4279–95.

52. Kim WS, Park BS, Sung JH, et al. Wound healing effect of adipose-derived stem cells: a critical role of secretory factors on human dermal fibroblasts. J Dermatol Sci 2007;48(1):15–24.

53. Rehman J, Traktuev D, Li J, et al. Secretion of angiogenic and antiapoptotic factors by human adipose stromal cells. Circulation 2004;109(10):1292–8.

54. Maeda K, Okubo K, Shimomura I, et al. Analysis of an expression profile of genes in the human adipose tissue. Gene 1997;190(2):227–35.

55. Chung HM, Won CH, Sung JH. Responses of adipose-derived stem cells during hypoxia: enhanced skin-regenerative potential. Expert Opin Biol Ther 2009;9(12):1499–508.

56. Park B, Jane KA, Sung J, et al. Adipose-derived stem cells and their secretory factors as a promising therapy for skin aging. Dermatol Surg 2008;34(10):1323–6.

57. Kim WS, Park BS, Park SH, et al. Antiwrinkle effect of adipose-derived stem cell: activation of dermal fibroblast by secretory factors. J Dermatol Sci 2009;53:96–102.

58. Kim WS, Park SH, Ahn SJ, et al. Whitening effect of adipose-derived stem cells: a critical role of TGF-beta 1. Biol Pharm Bull 2008;31(4):606–10.

59. Kim WS, Park BS, Kim HK, et al. Evidence supporting antioxidant action of adipose-derived stem cells: protection of human dermal fibroblasts from oxidative stress. J Dermatol Sci 2008;49(2):133–42.

60. Kim WS, Park BS, Sung JH. Protective role of adipose-derived stem cells and their soluble factors in photoaging. Arch Dermatol Res 2009;301(5):329–36.

61. Kim MH, Kim I, Kim SH, et al. Cryopreserved human adipogenic-differentiated pre-adipocytes: a potential new source for adipose tissue regeneration. Cytotherapy 2007;9(5):468–76.

62. Kern S, Eichler H, Stoeve J, et al. Comparative analysis of mesenchymal stem cells from bone marrow, umbilical cord blood, or adipose tissue. Stem Cells 2006;24(5):1294–301.

63. Wagner W, Wein F, Seckinger A, et al. Comparative characteristics of mesenchymal stem cells from human bone marrow, adipose tissue, and umbilical cord blood. Exp Hematol 2005;33(11):1402–16.

64. Gimble J, Guilak F. Adipose-derived adult stem cells: isolation, characterization, and differentiation potential. Cytotherapy 2003;5(5):362–9.

65. Guilak F, Lott KE, Awad HA, et al. Clonal analysis of the differentiation potential of human adipose-derived adult stem cells. J Cell Physiol 2006;206(1):229–37.

66. Lee RH, Kim B, Choi I, et al. Characterization and expression analysis of mesenchymal stem cells from human bone marrow and adipose tissue. Cell Physiol Biochem 2004;14(4–6):311–24.

67. Kinnaird T, Stabile E, Burnett MS, et al. Marrow-derived stromal cells express genes encoding a broad spectrum of arteriogenic cytokines and promote in vitro and in vivo arteriogenesis through paracrine mechanisms. Circ Res 2004;94(5):678–85.

68. Kratchmarova I, Kalume DE, Blagoev B, et al. A proteomic approach for identification of secreted proteins during the differentiation of 3T3-L1 preadipocytes to adipocytes. Mol Cell Proteomics 2002;1(3):213–22.

69. Schmid D, Schurch C, Blum P, et al. Plant stem cell extract for longevity of skin and hair. Seifen Ole Fette Wachse 2008;134:29–35.

70. Atiyeh BS, Ibrahim AE, Saad DA. Stem cell facelift: between reality and fiction. Aesthet Surg J 2013;33(3):334–8.

71. Byrne ME, Kidner CA, Martienssen RA. Plant stem cells: divergent pathways and common themes in shoots and roots. Curr Opin Genet Dev 2003;13:551–7.

Aesthetic Uses of the Botulinum Toxin

Andrew Dorizas, MD[a],*, Nils Krueger, PhD[a],
Neil S. Sadick, MD[a,b]

KEYWORDS

- Botulinum neurotoxin • Fillers • Perioral rhytides • Facial rhytides • Glabellar lines • BoNTA

KEY POINTS

- The cosmetic use of botulinum toxin (BoNT) is the most common cosmetic procedure performed in the world today.
- Thus far, the immunogenicity rates of onabotulinumtoxinA (BoNTA-ona) and incobotulinumtoxinA (BoNTA-inco) have been approximately 1%, whereas the immunogenicity rate for abobotulinum-toxinA (BoNTA-abo) is slightly higher, at 3%.
- Conversion ratios of 2.5:1.0 for BoNTA-abo: BoNTA-ona and 1:1 for BoNTA-inco: BoNTA-ona are widely accepted in the field.
- Common adverse events seen in the aesthetic use of the BoNT include swelling, localized bruising, headaches, injection site discomfort, excessive muscle weakness, and unintended paresis of adjacent muscles.
- BoNT has a wide array of cosmetic uses, including treatment of glabellar lines, chemical browlift, forehead wrinkles, periorbital, and perioral lines.
- The future formulations and applications of BoNTA will be plentiful, and are exciting to consider.

BACKGROUND

Aesthetic injection botulinum toxin (BoNT) is the most common cosmetic procedure performed in the world today.[1] BoNT has proven to be one of the most versatile agents used in the aesthetic field, and has also been used for numerous medical applications, including arm and leg spasticity, blepharospasm, cervical dystonia, strabismus, severe hyperhidrosis, chronic migraine, and overactive bladder, to name a few.[2]

Although the only U.S. Food and Drug Administration (FDA)–approved cosmetic indication for BoNT is the treatment of dynamic rhytides in the glabellar area, successful off-label uses of the products have been vast. Currently, the aesthetic market has multiple formulations available, and with the expected availability of more in the near future, it is important to understand that each

agent cannot be equivalent and, that differences and similarities exist between them. All products are synthesized by the same strain of anaerobic Clostridium botulinum, a gram-positive, rod-shaped anaerobic bacterium. The therapeutic preparations of botulinum neurotoxin however, vary in molecular weight, complexing proteins and excipients.

HISTORY OF BONT

C botulinum was discovered by professor of bacteriology, Emile Pierre van Ermengem, in 1895, after a botulism outbreak in a Belgian village.[2] The toxin itself, however, was not isolated until the 1920s.[1] Purification of the toxin was attempted by Dr Herman Sommer and colleagues at the University of California, San Francisco, but these attempts were not successful until Dr Edward Schantz

a Sadick Research Group, 911 Park Avenue, New York, NY 10075, USA; b Department of Dermatology, Weill Medical College of Cornell University, 1300 York Avenue, New York, NY 10065, USA
* Corresponding author.
E-mail address: adorizas@sadickdermatology.com

Dermatol Clin 32 (2014) 23–36
http://dx.doi.org/10.1016/j.det.2013.09.009

isolated a purified BoNT type A (BoNTA) in a crystalline form in the 1940s.

Approximately 30 years later, Dr Alan Scott, a surgeon at the Kettlewell Eye Research Institute in San Francisco, began testing BoNTA in monkeys as a potential therapy for strabismus. After successful treatments on monkeys, Dr Scott performed the first large-scale clinical trial using *onabotulinumtoxinA* (BoNTA-Ona) (Oculinum) to treat strabismus.[2–5] It was during this time that Dr Jean Carruthers noticed what was to become the future of BoNTA for aesthetic use: diminishing of wrinkles in the glabellar area. After Dr Scott's successful use of Oculinum, Allergan licensed his technology, named their product Botox, and received FDA approvals for both therapeutic and cosmetic indications, including strabismus and blepharospasm in 1989, cervical dystonia in 2000, glabellar lines in 2002, axillary hyperhidrosis in 2004, upper limb spasticity and chronic migraines in 2010, and urinary incontinence in 2011.[2,3] BoNT was the first microbial protein injection used to treat human disease.[6] In 1991, Speywood (now called Ispen) launched another BoNTA formulation based on abobotulinumtoxinA (BoNTA-abo), Dysport, for the treatment of blepharospasm, hemifacial spasm, and focal spasticity. Dysport was then approved for the treatment of glabellar lines in 2009. In 2000, Elan (now Solstice Neurosciences) brought its rimabotulinumtoxinB (BoNTB-rima)-based BoNT type B product Myobloc to market for the treatment of cervical dystonia, currently its only FDA-approved use. More recently, Merz Pharmaceuticals received regulatory approval for Xeomin, a product based on incobotulinumtoxinA (BoNTA-inco) for the treatment of focal dystonias, spasticity, and glabellar lines.

STRUCTURE AND MECHANISM OF ACTION

Seven serologically distinct BoNTs (BoNT types A, B, C, D, E, F, and G) are produced by various strains of *C botulinum*, *C butyricum*, and *C baratii* in nature. Only serotypes A and B are used therapeutically, with type A being the most neurotoxic.[7] The nontoxic accessory proteins are composed of hemagglutinin and nontoxin, nonhemagglutinin proteins, and spontaneously associate with the core neurotoxin after their cosynthesis by the bacteria.[8]

The size of the neurotoxin complexes is determined by serotype and accessory protein content. For example, type A clostridial strains produce complex sizes of 300, 500, and 900 kDa, whereas type B strains produce complexes of only 300 and 500 kDa.[9]

BoNT consists of 2 protein chains: a heavy chain (100 kDa) and a light chain (50 kDa), connected by a single disulfide bridge and noncovalent bonds. The heavy chain is made up of the binding and translocation domains. The light chain is the actual toxin itself. The binding domain attaches to the receptor on the neuronal end plate. The translocation domain causes endocytosis of the BoNT into the cytoplasm of the nerve. Simply, BoNT exerts its effects by inhibiting acetylcholine (Ach) release at the neuromuscular junction and autonomic nerve terminals. The effects of BoNT are nonpermanent. All formulations of BoNT inhibit exocytosis and Ach release without affecting Ach production or conduction of signaling along the nerve fiber.[7]

The process through which BoNT exerts its effect is dependent on a series of steps that begins with uptake of the toxin into the nerve terminal. BoNTA-ona, BoNTA-inco, and BoNTA-abo bind to the same cellular receptor synaptic vesicle protein 2 (SV-2), whereas BoNTB-rima binds to synaptotagmin II (Syt II) with great selectivity for these glycoproteins at the neuromuscular junction. Once internalized in the cell, the light chain dissociates from the heavy chain and cleaves one or more of the soluble *N*-ethylmaleimide–sensitive factor attachment receptors (SNAREs), which are part of the Ach transportation cascade and are required for docking of vesicles with the neural cell membrane in the release of Ach from the nerve terminal.[7] The light chain of each serotype of BoNT cleaves a different peptide bond, and no 2 serotypes do so at the same site. The substrate for BoNTA is a 25-kDa synaptosomal-associated protein (SNAP-25). BoNTB targets and cleaves vesicle-associated membrane proteins (synaptobrevins).[9]

Once the neuromuscular junction has been blocked by BoNT, binding sites for the toxin are decreased. As a result, repeated injection into an already denervated muscle is not as effective, because uptake into muscle is reduced. The neurotoxic effect of the neuromuscular junction is temporary. After injection, the effect is evident within 1 to 3 days. Maximal effect is seen approximately 2 weeks after the toxin is introduced, and then gradually starts to decline after approximately 3 months. Restoration of the neuromuscular junction is seen at 2 levels.[10] Axonal sprouting is a temporary recovery process, wherein new neuromuscular junctions develop around the blocked terminal. Once the original neuromuscular junction is restored, the sprouts are removed.

This inhibitory mechanism of action is also used in the treatment of hyperhidrosis. In addition to their effect on the neuromuscular junction, BoNTs have the ability to act on the innervated eccrine secretory cells. Through inhibiting the sympathetic fibers to sweat glands, where Ach is used as the neurotransmitter, BoNTs have been shown to effectively reduce sweat production.[11]

Other indications for the use of BoNT are based on the fact that sensory nerves release mediators of pain and inflammation, including substance P and cGRP (calcitonin gene-related peptide). Vesicles located at sensory nerve terminals also contain SNARE proteins that facilitate the release of these substances. In studies conducted using animals, BoNTA-ona has been shown to reduce cGRP. It has been suggested that blocking cGRP, glutamine, and substance P inhibits neurogenic inflammation and can ameliorate pain syndromes, such as migraine headache or psoriatic skin lesions.[9,12]

NONINTERCHANGEABILITY OF DIFFERENT FORMULATIONS

All BoNTA products cannot be generics, and each has a unique manufacturing process. BoNTA-ona, BoNTA-inco and BoNTA-abo are derived from a strain of *C botulinum* type A strain called *Hall strain*. BoNTB-rima is derived from a type B strain called *Bean strain*. BoNTA-ona is produced using a crystallization process that yields a homogenous formulation of 900-kDa complexes, whereas BoNTA-abo and BoNTB-rima are both manufactured with column chromatography. The process of BoNTA-abo production yields a heterogeneous

formulation of 300- and 500-kDa complexes, whereas BoNTB-rima manufacturing produces a homogenous mixture of complexes. The production of BoNTA-inco is distinctive, because the complexing proteins are separated and discarded from the neurotoxin during the manufacturing process in several purification steps. The resulting pure neurotoxin has a molecular weight of only 150 kDa. The excipient components of the vials, intentionally added substances that do not exert a therapeutic effect but may affect product delivery, vary among the formulations.[13]

All the products contain human serum albumin. Human serum albumin acts as a stabilizer of BoNT. As discussed by Pickett and Perrew,[13] the toxin is protected by the accessory proteins, which must dissociate for the core toxin to act. This dissociation occurs under physiologic conditions, including when the toxins are diluted with saline. Thus, the core toxin may be dissociated from the accessory proteins before injection. The amount of human serum albumin differs between the formulations.

The pH of the formulations depends on the pH of the preserved saline used and the ability of the excipients to buffer the solution. The number of units and the amount of core neurotoxin differs between the formulations. BoNTA-ona and BoNTA-inco are distributed in 100-U vials, BoNTA-abo in 300- and 500-U vials and BoNTB-rima in 2500-, 5000-, and 10,000-U vials. Therefore, the amount of neurotoxin injected depends on the dose of the product used (**Table 1**).

Table 1
Summary of commercially available botulinum toxin formulations

	Botox	Dysport	Xeomin	Myobloc
First approval	1989	1991	2011	2000
Serotype	A	A	A	B
Strain	Hall	Hall	Hall	Bean
Receptor/target	SV2/SNAP-25	SV2/SNAP-25	SV2/SNAP-25	Syt II/VAMP
Process	Crystallization	Chromatography	Chromatography	Chromatography
Complex size (kDa)	900	300	150	700
Uniformity	Homogeneous	Heterogeneous	Free neurotoxin	Homogeneous
Excipients	HSA Sodium chloride	HSA Lactose	HSA Sucrose	HSA Sodium chloride Sodium succinate
Stabilization	Vacuum drying	Lyophilization	Vacuum drying	Solution
Solubilization	Normal saline	Normal saline	Normal saline	N/A
Units per vial	100	300, 500	100	2500, 5000, 10,000

Abbreviations: HSA, human serum albumin; N/A, not applicable; SNAP-25, 25-kDa synaptosomal-associated protein; SV2, synaptic vesicle protein 2; Syt II, synaptotagmin II; VAMP, vesicle-associated membrane protein.

Data from Pickett A, Perrow K. Formulation composition of botulinum toxins in clinical use. J Drugs Dermatol 2010;9(9):1081–4; and Xeomin [package insert]. Greensboro (NC): Merz Pharmaceuticals, LLC; 2013.

As a result of the differences discussed, among others, it has been mandated that the product labeling include specific language that states that the unit and dose of each product are not interchangeable and cannot be simply converted between products.[2,14,15]

IMMUNOGENICITY

Because BoNT is a protein-based drug that is administered repeatedly for long-term effect, it is capable of triggering immunologic reactions and antibody formation. Various factors have an impact on its immunogenicity, such as prior exposure, manufacturing process, antigenic protein load, overall toxin dose administered, and presence of accessory proteins.[16,17]

Immunity in patients treated for indications requiring high doses, such as cervical dystonia, was as high as 20%.[18] In 1998 the manufacturer improved the purity of the BoNTA-ona formulation to decrease the amount of protein accompanying the toxin. Through decreasing the antigenic exposure, the immunity rates with repeated injections for cervical dystonia decreased and the purification did not alter dosing requirements.[10]

Because the protein content of BoNTA-inco is less than that of BoNTA-ona when comparing a 1-to-1 U dose equivalence, BoNTA-inco is expected to have a lower risk of immunogenicity. Although BoNTA-abo has a 2.5:1.0 equivalence ratio versus BoNTA-ona, the protein load is considerably smaller. Therefore, BoNTA-abo would also have a lower immunogenicity.[19,20]

However, currently no studies have directly compared antigenicity rates between currently available products. Factors that are thought to increase the incidence of antigenicity include increased treatment number and cumulative dose, frequent exposure, and genetic predisposition.[21–23] With these risk factors in mind, and given the increased doses used with BoNTA-abo and the shorter dosing interval, one might expect higher rates of antigenicity because of greater exposure to the toxin than when using BoNTA-ona. However, thus far, the immunogenicity rates of BoNTA-ona and BoNTA-inco have been around 1%, whereas the immunogenicity rate for BoNTA-abo is slightly higher at 3%.[16] BoNTA-inco has also been shown to induce an immunogenic response, which was established during the clinical trials performed in the United States. Twelve subjects developed neutralizing antibodies during the course of their trials.[19] The purification process for each BoNTA is different, and therefore experience with BoNTA-ona and immunogenicity cannot be used to estimate the risk of immunogenicity

with BoNTA-inco or BoNTA-abo. Overall, BoNTA products exhibit low clinically detectable levels of antibodies when compared with other approved biologic products, especially when used in low doses for aesthetic indications.[16]

CONTRAINDICATIONS AND ADVERSE EVENTS

Although generally treatments with BoNTA are considered safe, practitioners must be aware of the contraindications and adverse events and take the appropriate measures to minimize the risk. BoNT is contraindicated in any patient with known hypersensitivity to BoNT or any component of the formulation and in patients who have an active infection at the site to be injected.[14,15,24] Relative contraindications are in patients who are pregnant or nursing and anyone with a preexisting neuromuscular disease, such as myasthenia gravis and Eaton-Lambert syndrome. Although BoNT is classified as pregnancy category C in the United States, no teratogenicity has been reported as a result of women who inadvertently received up to 300 U of BoNTA during pregnancy.[21]

Common adverse events seen in the aesthetic use of the toxin include swelling, localized bruising, headaches, injection site discomfort, excessive muscle weakness, and unintended paresis of adjacent muscles.[14,15,24] Most of these adverse events have been comparable to those seen with placebo, as shown in several studies.[25–27] Avoiding anticoagulants or other blood-thinning supplements 2 weeks before the treatment can reduce the risk of bruising. Injection site discomfort can be avoided by using small-gauge needles and careful technique. If necessary, a topical anesthetic can be used or ice can be applied before the treatment. To avoid unintended muscle weakness, therapy should be initiated with lower doses and titrated upwards to achieve the desired effect. Lastly, using diluents containing preservatives has been shown to reduce patient discomfort during the injection.[28]

BoNT is among the most potent toxins in existence. Safety measures should be known and adhered to by all physicians, regardless of their experience. Proper patient selection and evaluation are crucial, along with precise injection technique. In most cases, adhering to the safety measures will avoid systemic exposure of the toxin.

HANDLING AND STORAGE

Studies have shown that BoNT formulations are not as fragile as suggested in the package instructions.

Prescribing information for BoNTA-ona, BoNTA-abo, BoNTA-inco, and BoNTB-rima state that each vial is for single use. BoNTB-rima is available in a ready-to-use form with no reconstitution necessary. Handling instructions state that vials should be refrigerated and used within 4 hours of reconstitution in the case of BoNTA-abo and BoNTB-rima, and within 24 hours of reconstitution in the case of BoNTA-ona and BoNTA-inco. BoNTA-inco, however, does not require refrigeration. Exposure to direct sunlight is thought to inactivate the toxin within 1 to 3 hours, and temperatures of 80°C to 100°C denature the toxin in approximately 30 and 10 minutes, respectively.[14,15,24]

Hexsel and colleagues[29] published a study that showed that the efficacy of BoNT was not compromised for up to 6 weeks after reconstitution. Similarly, a different study showed no contrast in the efficacy of freshly reconstituted BoNTA and BoNTA-ona that was reconstituted 2 weeks before being injected and then stored in either a freezer or a refrigerator. This study, and also one conducted by Sloop and colleagues,[30] showed that proper storage could be in either a freezer or a refrigerator.[31]

A recent animal study examined the effect of sustained agitation of BoNTA-ona for 6 weeks after reconstitution. The agitated BoNTA-ona was subsequently injected into mice to determine if it was still lethal (LD50). The study found no loss of efficacy in the vigorously agitated BoNTA-ona.[32] Additional studies have compared the efficacy of gently and vigorously reconstituted BoNTA-ona used for the treatment of rhytides in human subjects. These studies concluded that no loss of effect occurred with vigorous reconstitution.[33]

ONSET AND DURATION

Awareness with respect to expected time to relapse of a treated area after BoNT injections is vital in scheduling the subsequent appointment. It is generally accepted that the average duration of effect is between 3 and 4 months. A study conducted by Carruthers and colleagues[34] evaluated the efficacy of BoNTA-ona for the treatment of glabellar lines. The investigators determined that the rate of response at maximal frown lasted 3 months for most patients, and as long as 4 months in 25% of the patients, showing that 3- to 4-month intervals between injections is appropriate. Likewise, a study using BoNTA-abo with a 50-U dose versus placebo determined that the optimal timing for a second injection was between 3 and 4 months. Another study with more than 700 subjects treated with BoNTA-abo found a median duration of effect of 85 to 109 days.[26] One study showed a difference in response rate at 16 weeks between 2 different formulations; the relapse rate was 23% for BoNTA-ona and 40% for BoNTA-abo.[35] BoNTA-inco has been shown to have similar efficacy duration as BoNTA-ona, although more clinical studies are warranted for further comparison.[36,37]

A recent study of 45 patients using both patient and physician assessments of response after treatment of glabellar rhytides examined the onset of BoNTA-ona. Results showed that the mean time to response after treatment with a 20-U dose of BoNTA-ona was less than 2 days. In this study 48% of patients had onset on 1 day after injection and 87% of patients experienced a response by day 2.[38] Studies analyzing the onset of BoNTA-abo indicated that the mean onset time was 3 days, with effects seen in as early as 24 hours.[39]

BoNTB-rima has been associated with a faster onset but a shorter duration of action, with relapse times between 2 and 3 months.[40,41]

CONVERSION RATIOS

Although different formulations cannot be directly compared, knowing the approximate dose conversions between BoNT products is essential to incorporate them into practice, and for studies that seek to accurately compare these products. The conversion ratio of 2.5:1.0 (BoNTA-abo:BoNTA-ona) is widely accepted in the field. In an editorial commentary on the use of the 2 formulations for cervical dystonia, Poewe[42] stated that, based on clinical studies, the ratio of BoNTA-abo to BoNTA-ona should be no greater than 3.0:1.0. A study for the cosmetic use of BoNT used electromyographic activity to determine more precisely the dose conversion. This study enrolled 26 patients, each of whom was randomly assigned to receive BoNTA-abo and BoNTA-ona at a 3.0:1.0 ratio to each half of the frontalis muscle at 3 points of injection. Electromyographic activity was then measured at intervals as long as 20 weeks after the first injections. Results showed that at a 3.0:1.0 conversion ratio, the BoNTA-abo had a longer duration of effect. These results were interpreted as an indication that the true conversion ratio must be less than 3.0:1.0, because an accurate conversion ratio would have both formulations with equal duration of effect.[43] Lowe and colleagues[35] compared the duration of effect between BoNTA-abo and BoNTA-ona in the glabella using a dose ratio of 2.5:1.0. The study showed a greater duration of effect in patients treated with the 20-U dose of BoNTA-ona.

DIFFUSION

The toxin's ability to remain relatively localized at the site of injection is essential for the safety of BoNT treatments. Uncontrolled spread, diffusion, or migration of the toxin not only increases the risk of distal and systemic effects but also makes the aesthetic outcome unpredictable for the treating physician.

An often-cited study by Trinidade de Almeida and colleagues[44] compared the area of anhidrosis of each side of the forehead after injection of BoNTA-ona and BoNTA-abo to contrast their diffusion properties. Either side of each subject's forehead was randomized to receive either BoNTA-ona or BoNTA-abo at 2 injection points (medial and lateral). The side of the forehead randomized to BoNTA-ona received 3 U at each injection point. The alternate side was then randomized to receive an equal volume of injection of BoNTA-abo but with a dose ratio of 1.0:2.5, 1.0:3.0, or 1.0:4.0. An iodine and starch test across the forehead was used to highlight the areas of anhidrosis. The halos of anhidrosis could then be measured and compared. The important factor in this study is that the injections were kept at constant volume regardless of the dose ratio. The anhidrotic halo for BoNTA-abo was found to be larger at all dose ratios from week 1 to month 6 compared with the halos for BoNTA-ona.

Studies comparing BoNTA-ona and BoNTA-inco showed that the complex proteins in BoNTA-ona do not influence the diffusion profile.[45,46] BoNTB consistently showed the highest local and systemic diffusion properties. The B serotype not only produced a greater radius of toxin diffusion but also had a significantly higher number of associated side effects.[47,48] Brodsky and colleagues[49] summarize that neither molecular weight nor the presence of complexing proteins seem to affect diffusion, but properties intrinsic to the drug, accurate muscle selection, and dilution, volume, and dose injected are factors that influence diffusion.[50]

COSMETIC USES
Glabellar Lines

Treatment of the glabellar remains the only FDA-approved cosmetic use for BoNT. This treatment is by far the most common cosmetic use of BoNTA, and its efficacy has been shown in numerous clinical trials. The target site for the treatment is the procerus muscle and the corrugator supercilii muscle (**Fig. 1**). These muscles are responsible for depressing the medial brow. In an early dose-ranging study, Carruthers and

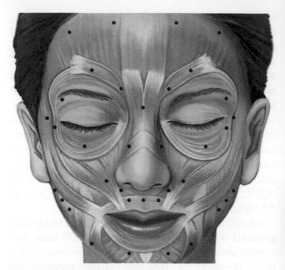

Fig. 1. BoNT injection points.

Carruthers[50] tested the safety, efficacy, and duration of response of 4 doses of BoNTA-ona on glabellar rhytides in men. The subjects were randomized to receive a total dose of 20, 40, 60, or 80 U of BoNTA-ona in the glabellar area. Seven injections points were used and the units were distributed evenly among the points. Results showed that increasing doses had more efficacy in reducing glabellar lines. They concluded that men with glabellar rhytides benefit from a starting dose of at least 40 U.[49]

In a similar study, Carruthers[28] examined the effect of 4 doses of BoNTA-ona in female subjects. In addition, an open-label arm of the trial evaluated the use of a 30-U dose in all subjects. Subjects were randomly administered 10, 20, 30, or 40 U. The investigators concluded that 20 U was an optimal dose for treating glabellar lines in woman, but that higher doses were not associated with an increase in adverse events and therefore can be administered if necessary.[28]

Frampton and Easthope[51] compared BoNTA-ona with placebo in 2 large clinical trials in 537 subjects with moderate to severe glabellar lines. Investigators and subjects both saw a clear improvement in the treatment group versus the control group throughout all the study visits. The efficacy of BoNTA-ona has been concluded in many publications.[36,52,53]

In a study[54] comparing the effects of BoNTA-ona versus BoNTA-inco in the treatment of glabellar frown lines, response rates were similar for both formulations at the same dose (1 U). Investigator assessment and high patient satisfaction rates confirmed high treatment success for both formulations at the same dose. Both formulations of the toxin (BoNTA-ona and BoNTA-inco) are generally administered at comparable doses for the same indications.[54]

International consensus recommendation for the treatment of glabellar lines with BoNTA-abo is 5 injection points, with 10 U injected per site (**Fig. 2**).[55] In addition to dynamic lines, lines present at rest may soften or be eliminated with BoNT to the glabellar region.[56]

Chemical Browlift

BoNT injections can lead to a desirable elevation in the resting position of the eyebrow. This technique will give the eye a more open appearance and a youthful look. Through paralyzing the lateral brow depressor (orbicularis oculi), the authors allow the frontalis muscle to elevate the brow without opposition. Treating the glabellar complex leads to a medial brow lift, and a lateral brow lift has also been shown.[57]

Frankel and Kamer[58] first noted the medial elevation and increase in interbrow distance with the use of BoNTA-ona for the treatment of glabellar lines. In a study of BoNTA-ona injected in the procerus and corrugator muscles in 30 subjects, they found that 32% of patients had a raise in medial eyebrow position, 48% had a higher eyebrow position in the midpupillary line, and 59% had an increase in the interbrow distance.

Chen and Frankel[59] discussed the various manipulations of the eyebrow position that can be achieved with BoNT. They note that slowly injecting BoNTA-ona at doses up to 10 U above the orbital rim may help avoid affecting the levator palpebrae muscle and causing an undesirable lid ptosis.

Maas and Kim[60] examined the effect of 5 to 10 U of BoNTA-ona or BoNTA-abo in 22 subjects injected into the lateral portion of the orbicularis oculi. Their study, and others, show statistical significant increases in the lateral brow height.[57,61]

In clinical practice the chemical browlift is more commonly performed in combination with other BoNT treatments for other target areas. When targeting the orbicularis oculi together with the glabella complex, a natural looking and aesthetically pleasing result can be achieved.

Forehead Wrinkles

Horizontal forehead lines occur when the frontalis muscle contracts to raise the eyebrows upward. The frontalis muscle has a rear belly and an anterior belly. The rear belly is continuous with and transitions to become the aponeurosis of the scalp via the tendinous galea aponeurotica. This transition point varies from person to person. Contraction of the rear belly does not cause a significant effect on the anterior belly of the frontalis muscle, and thus injections in the aponeurotic area have no clinical significance.[62]

Carruthers and colleagues[63] determined that BoNTA-ona can be used safely and effectively to treat forehead wrinkles. They found that the efficacy improves with higher doses (24 U) injected into the frontalis compared with lower doses (16 and 8 U). The consensus recommendations regarding use of BoNTA-ona in the upper face advise a range of 6 to 15 U in women. In men, the recommended dose is 6 to 15 U. The usual number of injections points is between 4 and 8.

International consensus recommends doses of 5 to 10 U of BoNTA-abo at 4 to 6 injection points for forehead lines, up to a total of 20 to 60 U.[55]

In a case series reporting on a man and a woman with forehead, glabellar, and periorbital lines injected with BoNT at 4-month intervals over a 7-year period[64] showed continued improvement in skin smoothening and effacement of nonreducible horizontal forehead lines. The investigators concluded that this showed evidence of ongoing dermal and epidermal remodeling, and that forehead lines can show long-term reduction when treated with BoNTA-ona injections. An assessment of wrinkle depth using silicone masks and multiphoton microscopy 3 weeks after injection with BoNTA-ona showed an objective improvement compared with baseline.[65]

When treating horizontal forehead lines, injections must be placed 1 to 2 cm above the orbital border to avoid eyebrow ptosis. The average target sites for forehead lines are between 5 and 10, depending on the patient. The points are generally in a V-shape or 2 horizontal lines approximately 1 cm apart. The lateral forehead should also be treated to avoid excessively arched eyebrows ("Spock" eyebrow) (**Fig. 3**).[66]

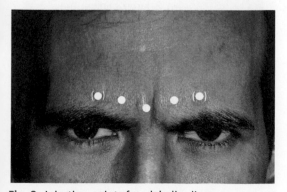

Fig. 2. Injection points for glabellar lines.

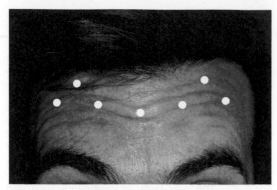

Fig. 3. Injection points for forehead wrinkles.

Periorbital Lines

Periorbital lines or crow's feet are among the most popular treatment sites for BoNT. These dynamic lateral canthal lines appear when smiling, and are not to be confused with the static lateral canthal lines that are caused by photoaging. Static lines are more resistant to BoNT treatments and require additional procedure to be corrected, including laser resurfacing.

Consensus data, clinical studies, and experience support that the usual number of injection points for crow's feet is 2 to 5 (average of 3) per side, and that dosing of BoNTA-ona and BoNTA-inco ranges from 10 to 30 U for women and 20 to 30 U for men (**Fig. 4**). For BoNTA-abo, the recommended dosing is 20 to 60 U divided among 3 injection points per side.[63] The injections should be at least 1.0 to 1.5 cm from the external orbital rim to avoid any paralysis of the palpebral portion of the orbicularis oculi muscle.[67]

A study of 162 patients evaluated the treatment of crow's feet with doses of 3, 6, 12, and 18 U. The investigators found that the optimal dose was 12 U because it was more effective than the smaller doses, but they noted no significant difference between the 12- and 18-U doses.[68] A study by Levy and colleagues[69] showed that wrinkles in the periorbital area were significantly improved for up to 6 months after injection of the crow's feet with 12 U of BoNTA-ona on each side.

Adverse events that may occur with treatment of the crow's feet include periorbital hematoma, dry eyes, eyelid ptosis, and mouth droop. The zygomaticus major muscle is located nearby and, as a precaution, the injector should never inject beneath the zygoma to avoid paralyzing it. Using the minimal injection dose and correcting injection target sites are essential to avoid and adverse events.[70]

Bunny Lines

Bunny lines are multiple dynamic rhytides located on the upper nasal dorsum that result from the contraction of the transverse nasalis muscle with smiling. These lines can become more prominent after BoNT treatment in the glabella and periorbital region. A single injection of 2 to 4 U of BoNTA-ona or 5 to 10 U of BoNTA-abo should be injected on each side about 1 cm superior to the alar grove.[71] Injecting into the levator labii superioris or alaeque nasi can lead to upper lip ptosis (**Fig. 5**).

Gummy Smile

An excessive gingival display or gummy smile is defined as gingival exposure greater than 2.0 mm above the dental line with smiling. This condition may be considered aesthetically unappealing and is more common in women. In a study involving 52 subjects, Sucupira and Abramovitz[72] injected

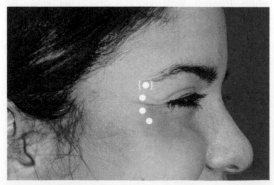

Fig. 4. Injection points for crow's feet.

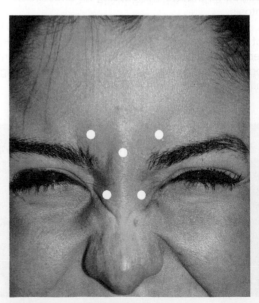

Fig. 5. Injection points for bunny lines.

BoNTA-ona to the levator labii superioris alaeque nasi muscle. The average dose was 1.95 U per side. The average gingival display was 3.62 mm before treatment, and 0.58 mm after treatment. The results showed that injecting just the levator labii superioris can be effective in correcting excessive gingival display.

Polo[73] documented the treatment of 12 women with gummy smile. Each elevator muscle was injected with variable dosing in 3 phases. He used 3 injection points on each side, injecting 2.5 U of BoNTA-ona into the levator labii superioris, the junction of the levator labii superioris, and the zygomaticus minor, and 1.5 U into the orbicularis oris at a point 2 to 3 mm below the nares and 2 to 3 mm away from midline.

In a study of 16 patients, Mazzuco and Hexsel[74] categorized the type of gummy visibility present, and then based the treatment on the muscles that were responsible for each type. Subjects were categorized into 4 groups: anterior gummy show defined as greater than 3 mm of gum exposure in the area between the canine teeth; posterior gummy show defined as normal anterior exposure but posterior to the canines; greater than 3 mm of gingival display mixed with gum exposure both anteriorly and posteriorly; and lastly, asymmetric gummy show. Subjects with anterior gummy show were treated with 5.0 U of BoNTA-abo into the levator labii superioris alaeque nasi bilaterally, whereas subjects with posterior gummy smile were given injections of 2.5 U into the zygomaticus major and 2.5 U into the zygomaticus minor. Subjects in the mixed group were treated in all 3 areas, and subjects in the asymmetric group were treated according to the asymmetry. These authors supported the principle that lower dilution volumes should be used for this indication given the proximity to important functional muscles. Suggested doses for BoNTA-ona, BoNTA-inco are 2.0 to 5.0 U and 5.0 to 15.0 U for BoNTA-abo.

Perioral Lines

Perioral lines, or lipstick lines, are vertical rhytides projecting in a perpendicular fashion from the vermillion border of the lips. Movements of the orbicularis oris muscle, such as puckering, and smoking, photoaging, and hereditary factors contribute to the formation of these rhytides.[75,76] In the upper lip, 4 injection points are recommended, and 2 in the lower lip. The injection points should be at the vermillion border at least 1.5 cm away from the oral commissures. Because this is a very delicate area that can lead to functional impairment of the lips (eg, eating, drinking,

drooling), administering the minimum dose is recommended (0.5 U of BoNTA-ona and BoNTA-inco and 1.0 U of BoNTA-abo) and then increased on a case-by-case basis.

Additionally, other treatment modalities, including laser resurfacing and injectable fillers, may be required for full correction. This location should not be injected in patients who use their mouth to play musical instruments, because these patients rely on the full function of the orbicularis oris.[2] Consensus guidelines on the topic of perioral rhytides include similar recommendations, including using low doses and avoiding central and lateral injections points that may flatten the cupid's bow, and lead to drooling or drooping, respectively.[77] These guidelines state that it is safer to keep injections within 5 mm of the vermillion border. Ice may be used as an anesthetic before injections in this more sensitive area.

Dimpled Chin

The dimpling of the chin, or peau d'orange (orange peel) appearance, is caused by a combination of loss of volume and contraction of the mentalis muscle.[78] A combination of BoNT and dermal fillers is recommended to achieve optimal results. Consensus recommendations state that generally 1 injection point per side is needed just below the tip of the chin close to the mandibular bone.[68] A typical dose is 5 to 10 U of BoNTA-ona and BoNTA-inco and 10 to 20 U of BoNTA-abo; however, men may require higher doses. Lowe and colleagues[68] recommended careful avoidance of an injection point that is too close to the lips, which could lead to loss of function of the lip depressors. Furthermore, when treating the dimpled chin along with the oral commissures, the dose must be decreased accordingly to avoid overtreatment.[63]

Marionette Lines

The marionette lines, or melomental folds, are also best treated with a combination approach of BoNT and dermal fillers.

The depressor anguli oris contributes to depressing the mouth and draw it laterally, causing a sad face appearance. A recent retrospective analysis of 60 patients treated with BoNT found that 10% to 20% received injections into the depressor anguli oris.[78] The injection should be at the level of the mandible to avoid affecting the depressor labii inferioris muscle. A dose of 3 to 5 U of BoNTA-ona and BoNTA-inco or 5 to 10 U BoNTA-abo is recommended at the posterior portion of the depressor anguli oris near the anterior portion of the masseter.[79]

Masseter

The appearance of a wide jaw, which can be undesirable in many cases, is caused by the hypertrophy of the masseter muscle. BoNT injections to treat a hypertrophic masseter are not the most common indication, but are seen more often in Asians. The paralysis of the muscle leads to a smoother and slimmer appearance. Ahn and colleagues[80] treated 19 Asian patients with injections of BoNTA-ona at the inferior border of the masseter. The initial dose was 25 U per side, and then at 1-week follow-up an additional 25-U dose was administered if needed; 3 of the patients required a third dose. They found that maximum correction occurred at 1 to 2 months, and reinjection was required at 6 to 8 months. A dosing study evaluated treatment doses of 10, 20, and 30 U of BoNTA-ona in 22 patients.[81] The investigators used ultrasonographic imaging to compare the thickness of the masseter muscles before and after injection, and concluded that the optimal dose was 20 U. Results were maintained for 6 months after treatment.

In a study evaluating the treatment of masseter hypertrophy in non-Asian, Western populations, Liew and Dar[82] used doses of 25 to 30 U of BoNTA-ona on each side and compared the results with those of previously treated Asian patients. Results showed that BoNTA-ona injections were successful in treating masseter hypertrophy in Western patients. Similar to the experiences of other investigators, they cautioned about careful placement of the injections. They recommended that the injection point should be below the sigmoid notch, approximately 1 cm above the mandibular angle border.[80] They noted few cases of difficulty with eating that lasted 4 weeks. Improvement in the lower face resulted in prominence of the cheek bones in the Western population, an effect that is typically very desirable. Similarly, Choi and Park found that among 45 patients who were injected with 25 to 30 U of BoNTA-ona, most were satisfied. However, most patients also experienced difficulty with mastication, commonly followed by muscle aching. To avoid any side effects, it is advisable to begin treatment with smaller doses and re-treat as needed.[83,84]

Several studies have noted the longer duration of effect when treating masseter hypertrophy. This finding is probably because the muscle hypertrophy is caused by the excessive muscle use in these subjects, which is mitigated after the BoNT injection. Regaining the baseline muscle mass after attenuated contraction takes longer than simply regaining function.[71,72]

Platysmal Bands

Contraction of the platysma muscle can result in prominent vertical bands in patients who are thin. Horizontal neck lines can also be caused by muscle activity or skin laxity. BoNTA can be a safe and effective treatment to reduce both the platysmal bands and the horizontal lines caused by muscle activity. Careful patient selection is important when evaluating platysmal band treatment with BoNTA. The ideal patient should have good skin elasticity in the neck and little or no fat.[63,68]

The injection points should be superficially into each platysmal band, beginning below the jaw line and spacing each injection approximately 2 cm apart. A total of 3 to 5 injections per side is recommended with 2 to 4 U of BoNTA-ona and BoNTA-inco and 5 to 10 U of BoNTA-abo.[2,78]

The greatest risk associated with injection into the platysmal bands is dysphagia or weakening of the muscles of the neck responsible for holding the head up. The maximum recommended dose should not be exceeded to avoid causing any side effects (40–60 U of BoNTA-ona and BoNTA-inco and 100 U of BoNTA-abo).[68]

Another interesting cosmetic use of BoNT injected into the platysma is for the technique called the Nefertiti lift. Levy[85] published an article describing a method of contouring the jawline with BoNT. His method is to treat platysma fibers along the jawline laterally from the nasolabial fold up to the mandibular angle and into the posterior platysmal band. A total of 130 patients were injected with a total dose of 20 U of BoNTA-ona, distributed in 2 to 3 U per injection site. The study concluded that this technique was successful in creating a mini-lift of the jawline in patients who wanted an alternative to invasive surgical correction.

INDICATIONS IN MEDICAL DERMATOLOGY

Similar to the facial aesthetic use of BoNT, its use in medical dermatology has also grown impressively. BoNTA-ona was approved for the use of axillary hyperhidrosis, and its use has expanded into other dermatologic uses of BoNT. Some off-label uses include treatment of palmar and plantar hyperhidrosis, Raynaud disease, dyshidrotic eczema, lichen simplex, Hailey-Hailey disease, piloleiomyomas and leiomyomas, anal fissures, and inverse psoriasis.[86–94]

ON THE HORIZON

Other BoNT products that have been developed or are currently in development are aiming to improve on the toxin formulations currently available.

A topical gel containing BoNTA, RT001 (Revance Therapeutics, Newark, CA, USA), is currently under development for the treatment of crow's feet. The topical get contains both the toxin and a peptide that helps facilitate transport through the skin.

Two controlled studies evaluating the efficacy of RT001, involving 126 patients overall, showed clinically relevant improvement in lateral canthal line severity in 9 of 10 patients. They found that 50% of subjects had a 2-point improvement on the severity scale, and 9 of 10 patients had a 1-point improvement versus placebo, which showed 0% and 15% improvement, respectively. No increase was seen in adverse events compared with placebo.[95,96] PurTox (Mentor Corporation, Santa Barbara, CA, USA) will be the second BoNTA formulation that does not have any complexing proteins. Three phase III clinical trials with more than 600 subjects have been conducted to evaluate the efficacy and safety of PurTox for the treatment of glabellar lines. However, no data have yet been published.

Also on the horizon is a new toxin-free modality of relaxing a specific target muscle. The Iovera device (Myoscience, Redwood City, CA, USA) delivers compressed liquid nitrous oxide to a close-ended 27-gauge, 6-mm-long, 3-needle probe that cools the temporal branch of the facial nerve. The resulting temperature of –60° C temporarily inhibits motor nerve conduction, resulting in inhibition of voluntary contraction of the muscle. Recently published data from a preclinical study reveal demyelination and axonal degeneration 2 weeks posttreatment, followed by complete axonal regeneration and remyelination after 16 weeks.[97] The device has been approved in Canada and the European Union for the treatment of dynamic facial wrinkles.

SUMMARY

Injection of BoNT is the most common cosmetic procedure performed in the United States today.[1] From its incidental discovery to its numerous medical and aesthetic uses, BoNT has a wide potential. Since its approval for cosmetic use in the glabellar area in 2002, the applications of BoNT have expanded to the entire face and the neck. With the increasing number of available products, the noninterchangeability between products will make it important to determine how these products should be evaluated in studies that seek to compare dosing, efficacy, and longevity. Additional research is warranted to resolve the outstanding controversies surrounding antibody formation, diffusion, efficacy, and duration of effect of the different formulations. As combination therapies with concurrent use of BoNTA, fillers, and energy-based devices are becoming more common in clinical practice, further studies are needed to evaluate the combinability of these treatments for facial rejuvenation.

REFERENCES

1. Carruthers J, Carruthers A. The evolution of botulinum neurotoxin type A for cosmetic applications. J Cosmet Laser Ther 2007;9(3):186–92.
2. Botox [package insert]. Irvine (CA): Allergan, Inc; 2013.
3. van Ermengem E. Classics in infectious diseases. A new anaerobic bacillus and its relation to botulism. E. van Ermengem. Originally published as "Ueber einen neuen anaeroben Bacillus und seine Beziehungen zum Botulismus" in Zeitschrift fur Hygiene und Infektionskrankheiten 1897;26:1-56. Rev Infect Dis 1979;1(4):701–19.
4. Carruthers JD, Carruthers JA. Treatment of glabellar frown lines with C. botulinum-A exotoxin. J Dermatol Surg Oncol 1992;18:17–21.
5. Simpson LL. The origin, structure, and pharmacological activity of botulinum toxin. Pharmacol Rev 1981;33:155–88.
6. Erbguth FJ. Historical notes on botulism, Clostridium botulinum, botulinum toxin and the idea of the therapeutic use of the toxin. Mov Disord 2004; 19(Suppl 8):s2–6.
7. Aoki KR. Pharmacology and immunology of botulinum neurotoxins. Int Ophthalmol Clin 2005;45(3): 25–37.
8. Inoue K, Fujinaga Y, Watanabe T, et al. Molecular composition of clostridium botulinum type A progenitor toxins. Infect Immun 1996;64:1589–94.
9. Wenzel RG. Pharmacology of botulinum neurotoxin serotype A. Am J Health Syst Pharm 2004; 61(Suppl 6):S5–10.
10. Chen JJ, Dashtipour K. Abo-, inco-, ona-, and rimabotulinum toxins in clinical therapy: a primer. Pharmacotherapy 2013;33(3):304–18.
11. Bhidayasiri R, Truong DD. Evidence for effectiveness of botulinum toxin for hyperhidrosis. J Neural Transm 2008;115:641–5.
12. Ward NL, Kavlick KD, Diaconu D, et al. Botulinum neurotoxin A decreases infiltrating cutaneous lymphocytes and improves acanthosis in the KC-Tie2 mouse model. J Invest Dermatol 2012;132(7): 1927–30.
13. Pickett A, Perrow K. Formulation composition of botulinum toxins in clinical use. J Drugs Dermatol 2010;9(9):1081–4.
14. Xeomin [package insert]. Greensboro (NC): Merz Pharmaceuticals, LLC; 2013.
15. Dysport [package insert]. Scottsdale (AZ): Medicis Aesthetics Inc; 2012.

16. Naumann M, Boo LM, Ackerman AH, et al. Immunogenicity of botulinum toxins. J Neural Transm 2013;120(2):275–90.

17. Atassi MZ. Basic immunological aspects of botulinum toxin therapy [review]. Mov Disord 2004; 19(Suppl 8):S68–84.

18. Sattler G. Current and future botulinum neurotoxin type A preparations in aesthetics: a literature review. J Drugs Dermatol 2010;9:1065–71.

19. Frevert J. Content of botulinum neurotoxin in Botox®/Vistabel®, Dysport®/Azzalure®, and Xeomin®/Bocouture®. Drugs R D 2010;10(2):67–73.

20. Frevert J, Dressler D. Complexing proteins in botulinum toxin type A drugs: a help or a hindrance? Biologics 2010;4:325–32.

21. Li Yim JF, Weir CR. Botulinum toxin and pregnancy—a cautionary tale. Strabismus 2010;18(2): 65–6.

22. Schellekens H. Immunogenicity of therapeutic proteins: clinical implications and future prospects. Clin Ther 2002;24(11):1720–40.

23. Carruthers A, Kane MA, Flynn TC, et al. The convergence of medicine and neurotoxins: a focus on botulinum toxin type A and its application in aesthetic medicine—a global, evidence-based botulinum toxin consensus education initiative: part I: botulinum toxin in clinical and cosmetic practice. Dermatol Surg 2013;39:493–509.

24. BOTOX [package insert]. Irvine (CA): Allergan, Inc; 2011.

25. Gadhia K, Whimsley AD. Facial aesthetics: is botulinum toxin treatment effective and safe? A systemic review of randomized controlled trials. Br Dent J 2009;207(5):E9.

26. Brin MF, Boodhoo TI, Pogoda JM, et al. Safety and tolerability of onabotulinumtoxinA in the treatment of facial lines: a meta-analysis of individual patient data from global clinical registration studies in 1678 participants. J Am Acad Dermatol 2009; 61(6):961–70.

27. Cote TR, Mohan AK, Polder JA, et al. Botulinum toxin type A injections: adverse events reported to the US Food and Drug Administration in therapeutic and cosmetic cases. J Am Acad Dermatol 2005;53(3):407–15.

28. Carruthers J, Fournier N, Kerscher M, et al. The convergence of medicine and neurotoxins: a focus on botulinum toxin type A and its application in aesthetic medicine—a global, evidence-based botulinum toxin consensus education initiative: part II: incorporating botulinum toxin into aesthetic clinical practice. Dermatol Surg 2013;39(3 Pt 2):510–25.

29. Hexsel DM, De Almeida AT, Rutowitsch M, et al. Multicenter, double-blind study of the efficacy of injections with botulinum toxin type A reconstituted up to six consecutive weeks before application. Dermatol Surg 2003;29:523–9.

30. Sloop RR, Cole BA, Escutin RO. Reconstituted botulinum toxin type A does not lose potency in humans if it is refrozen or refrigerated for 2 weeks before use. Neurology 1997;48:249–53.

31. Yang GC, Chiu RJ, Gillman GS. Questioning the need to use Botox (OnabotulinumtoxinA) within 4 hours of reconstitution: a study of fresh vs 2-week-old Botox (OnabotulinumtoxinA). Arch Facial Plast Surg 2008;10:273–9.

32. Shome D, Nair AH, Kapoor R, et al. Botulinum toxin A: is it really that fragile a molecule? Dermatol Surg 2010;36:2106–10.

33. Kazim NA, Black EH. Botox: shaken, not stirred. Ophthal Plast Reconstr Surg 2008;24(1):10–2.

34. Carruthers A, Carruthers J, Said S. Dose-ranging study of botulinum toxin type A in the treatment of glabellar rhytids in females. Dermatol Surg 2005; 31(4):414–22.

35. Lowe P, Patnaik R, Lowe N. Comparison of two formulations of botulinum toxin type A for the treatment of glabellar lines: a double-blind, randomized study. J Am Acad Dermatol 2006;55(6):975–80.

36. Prager W, Bee EK, Havermann I, et al. Onset, longevity, and patient satisfaction with incobotulinumtoxinA for the treatment of glabellar frown lines: a single-arm, prospective clinical study. Clin Interv Aging 2013;8:449–56.

37. Chundury RV, Couch SM, Holds JB. Comparison of preferences between onabotulinumtoxinA (Botox) and incobotulinumtoxinA (Xeomin) in the treatment of benign essential blepharospasm. Ophthal Plast Reconstr Surg 2013;29(3):205–7.

38. Beer KR, Boyd C, Patel RK, et al. Rapid onset of response and patient-reported outcomes after OnabotulinumtoxinA treatment of moderate-to-severe glabellar lines. J Drugs Dermatol 2011; 10(1):39–44.

39. Baumann L, Brandt FS, Kane MA, et al. An analysis of efficacy data from four phase III studies of botulinum neurotoxin type A-ABO for the treatment of glabellar lines. Aesthet Surg J 2009;29(Suppl 6): S57–65.

40. Flynn TC. Botulinum toxin: examining duration of effect in facial aesthetic applications. Am J Clin Dermatol 2010;11(3):189–99.

41. Sadick NS, Matarasso SL. Comparison of botulinum toxins A and B in the treatment of facial rhytides. Dermatol Clin 2004;22(2):221–6.

42. Poewe W. Respective potencies of Botox and Dysport: a double blind, randomized, crossover study in cervical dystonia—editorial commentary. J Neurol Neurosurg Psychiatry 2002;72:430.

43. Karsai S, Adrian R, Hammes S, et al. A randomized double-blind study of the effect of Botox and Dysport/Reloxin on forehead wrinkles and electromyographic activity. Arch Dermatol 2007;1143(11): 1447–9.

44. Trinidade de Almeida AR, Marques E, De Almeida J, et al. Pilot study comparing the diffusion of two formulations of botulinum toxin type A in patients with forehead hyperhidrosis. Dermatol Surg 2007;33(Suppl 1):S37–43.

45. Roggenkämper P, Jost WH, Bihari K, et al, NT 201 Blepharospasm Study Team. Efficacy and safety of a new botulinum toxin type A free of complexing proteins in the treatment of blepharospasm. J Neural Transm 2006;113(3):303–12.

46. Benecke R, Jost WH, Kanovsky P, et al. A new botulinum toxin type A free of complexing proteins for treatment of cervical dystonia. Neurology 2005; 64(11):1949–51.

47. Comella CL, Jankovic J, Shannon KM, et al, Dystonia Study Group. Comparison of botulinum toxin serotypes A and B for the treatment of cervical dystonia. Neurology 2005;65(9):1423–9.

48. Pappert EJ, Germanson T, Myobloc/Neurobloc European Cervical Dystonia Study Group. Botulinum toxin type B vs. type A in toxin-naïve patients with cervical dystonia: randomized, double-blind, noninferiority trial. Mov Disord 2008;23(4):510–7.

49. Brodsky MA, Swope DM, Grimes D. Diffusion of botulinum toxins. Tremor Other Hyperkinet Mov (N Y) 2012;2. pii:tre-02-85-417-1.

50. Carruthers A, Carruthers J. Prospective, double-blind, randomized, parallel-group, dose-ranging study of botulinum toxin type A in men with glabellar rhytids. Dermatol Surg 2005;31(10):1297–303.

51. Frampton JE, Easthope SE. Botulinum toxin A (Botox Cosmetic): a review of its use in the treatment of glabellar frown lines. Am J Clin Dermatol 2003;4(10):709–25.

52. Keen M, Blitzer A, Aviv J, et al. Botulinum toxin A for hyperkinetic facial lines: results of a double-blind, placebo-controlled study. Plast Reconstr Surg 1994;94(1):94–9.

53. Rzany B, Dill-Müller D, Grablowitz D, et al, German-Austrian Retrospective Study Group. Repeated botulinum toxin A injections for the treatment of lines in the upper face: a retrospective study of 4,103 treatments in 945 patients. Dermatol Surg 2007;33:S18–25.

54. Sattler G, Callander MJ, Grablowitz D, et al. Noninferiority of incobotulinumtoxinA, free from complexing proteins, compared with another botulinum toxin type A in the treatment of glabellar frown lines. Dermatol Surg 2010;36(Suppl 4):2146–54.

55. Ascher B, Talarico S, Cassuto D, et al. International consensus recommendations on the aesthetic usage of botulinum toxin type A (Speywood Unit)—part I: upper facial wrinkles. J Eur Acad Dermatol Venereol 2010;24(11):1278–84.

56. Carruthers A, Carruthers J, Lei X, et al. OnabotulinumtoxinA treatment of glabellar lines in repose. Dermatol Surg 2010;36:2168–71.

57. Carruthers A, Carruthers J. Eyebrow height after botulinum toxin type A to the glabella. Dermatol Surg 2007;33(1 Spec No):S26–31.

58. Frankel AS, Kamer FM. Chemical browlift. Arch Otolaryngol Head Neck Surg 1998;124(3):321–3.

59. Chen AH, Frankel AS. Altering brow contour with botulinum toxin. Facial Plast Surg Clin North Am 2003;11(4):457–64.

60. Maas CS, Kim EJ. Temporal brow lift using botulinum toxin A: an update. Plast Reconstr Surg 2003;112(Suppl 5):109S–12S.

61. Ahn MS, Catten M, Maas CS. Temporal brow lift using botulinum toxin A. Plast Reconstr Surg 2000; 105(3):1129–35.

62. Tamura BM. Standardization of muscle site for BTX injection in the frontal and glabellar regions. In: Hexsel S, Trindade de Almeida A, editors. Cosmetic use of botulinum toxin. Porto Alegre (Brazil): AGE Editoria; 2002. p. 145–8.

63. Carruthers JD, Glogau RG, Blizter A, et al. Advances in facial rejuvenation: botulinum toxin type A, hyaluronic acid dermal fillers and combination therapies—consensus recommendations. Plast Reconstr Surg 2008;121(Suppl 5):6S–30S.

64. Bowler PJ. Dermal and epidermal remodeling using botulinum toxin type A for facial, non-reducible, hyperkinetic lines: two case studies. J Cosmet Dermatol 2008;7(3):241–4.

65. Branford OA, Dann SC, Grobbelaar AO. The quantitative assessment of wrinkle depth: turning the microscope on botulinum toxin type A. Ann Plast Surg 2010;65(3):285–93.

66. Fagien S, Raspaldo H. Facial rejuvenation with botulinum neurotoxin: an anatomical and experimental perspective. J Cosmet Laser Ther 2007;9(Suppl 1): 23–31.

67. Ascher B, Talarico S, Cassuto D, et al. International consensus recommendations on the aesthetic usage of botulinum toxin type A (Speywood Unit)—part II: wrinkles on the middle and lower face, neck and chest. J Eur Acad Dermatol Venereol 2010;24(11):1285–95.

68. Lowe NJ, Ascher B, Heckmann M, et al. Double-blind, randomized, placebo-controlled, dose-response study of the safety and efficacy of botulinum toxin type A in subjects with crow's feet. Dermatol Surg 2005;31(3):257–62.

69. Levy JL, Servant JJ, Jouve E. Botulinum toxin A: a 9-month clinical and 3D in vivo profilometric crow's feet wrinkle formation study. J Cosmet Laser Ther 2004;6:16–20.

70. Klein AW. Contraindications and complications with the use of botulinum toxin. Clin Dermatol 2004; 22(1):66–75.

71. Carruthers J, Carruthers A. Aesthetic botulinum A toxin in the mid and lower face and neck. Dermatol Surg 2003;29(5):468–76.

72. Sucupira E, Abramovitz A. A simplified method for smile enhancement: botulinum toxin injection for gummy smile. Plast Reconstr Surg 2012;130(3):726–8.

73. Polo M. Botulinum toxin type A in the treatment of excessive gingival display. Am J Orthod Dentofacial Orthop 2005;127(2):214–8.

74. Mazzuco R, Hexsel D. Gummy smile and botulinum toxin: a new approach based on the gingival exposure area. J Am Acad Dermatol 2010;63(6): 1042–51.

75. Hexsel C, Hexsel D, Porto MD, et al. Botulinum toxin type A for aging face and aesthetic uses. Dermatol Ther 2011;24(1):54–61.

76. Semchyshyn N, Sengelmann RD. Botulinum toxin A treatment of perioral rhytides. Dermatol Surg 2003; 29(5):490–5.

77. Carruthers J, Fagien S, Matarasso SL, Botox Consensus Group. Consensus recommendations on the use of botulinum toxin type A in facial aesthetics. Plast Reconstr Surg 2004;114(Suppl 6): 1S–22S.

78. Sepehr A, Chauhan N, Alexander AJ, et al. Botulinum toxin type A for facial rejuvenation: treatment evolution and patient satisfaction. Aesthetic Plast Surg 2010;34(5):583–6.

79. Carruthers J, Carruthers A. Aesthetic uses of botulinum toxin A in the periocular region and mid and lower face. Operat Tech Otolaryngol Head Neck Surg 2004;15(2):134–8.

80. Ahn J, Horn C, Blitzer A. Botulinum toxin for masseter reduction in Asian patients. Arch Facial Plast Surg 2004;6(3):188–91.

81. Choe SW, Cho WI, Lee CK, et al. Effects of botulinum toxin type a on contouring of the lower face. Dermatol Surg 2005;11(5):502–8.

82. Liew S, Dar A. Nonsurgical reshaping of the lower face. Aesthet Surg J 2008;28(3):251–7.

83. Choi JH, Park SW, Chung HY, et al. Incidental aggravation of venous malformation after botulinum toxin type a injection for reducing benign masseteric hypertrophy. Dermatol Surg 2010;36: 2188–92.

84. Carruthers J, Carruthers A. Botox use in the mid and lower face and neck. Semin Cutan Med Surg 2001;20(2):85–92.

85. Levy PM. The 'Nefertiti lift': a new technique for specific re-contouring of the jawline. J Cosmet Laser Ther 2007;9(4):249–52.

86. Togel B, Greve B, Raulin C. Current therapeutic strategies for hyperhidrosis: a review. Eur J Dermatol 2002;12(3):219–23.

87. Fregene A, Ditmars D, Siddiqui A. Botulinum toxin type a: a treatment option for digital ischemia in patients with Raynaud's phenomenon. J Hand Surg Am 2009;34(3):446–52.

88. Bakke M, Max TN, Bardow A, et al. Treatment of gustatory sweating with low-dose botulinum toxin a: a case report. Acta Odontol Scand 2006;64(3): 129–33.

89. Swartling C, Naver H, Lindberg M, et al. Treatment of dyshidrotic hand dermatitis with intradermal botulinum toxin. J Am Acad Dermatol 2002; 47(5):667–71.

90. Koeyers WJ, Van Der Geer S, Krekels G. Botulinum toxin type a as an adjuvant treatment modality for extensive Hailey-Hailey disease. J Dermatolog Treat 2008;19(4):251–4.

91. Onder M, Adisen E. A new indication of botulinum toxin: leiomyoma-related pain. J Am Acad Dermatol 2009;60(2):325–8.

92. Brisinda G, Cadeddu F, Brandara F, et al. Randomized clinical trial comparing botulinum toxin injections with 0.2 percent nitroglycerin ointment for chronic anal fissure. Br J Surg 2007;94(2):162–7.

93. Zanchi M, Favot F, Bizzarini M, et al. Botulinum toxin type A for the treatment of inverse psoriasis. J Eur Acad Dermatol Venereol 2008;22(4):431–6.

94. Heckmann M, Heyer G, Brunner B, et al. Botulinum toxin type A injection in the treatment of lichen simplex: an open pilot study. J Am Acad Dermatol 2002;46(4):617–9.

95. Brandt F, O'Connell C, Cazzaniga A, et al. Efficacy and safety evaluation of a novel botulinum toxin topical gel for the treatment of moderate to severe lateral canthal lines. Dermatol Surg 2010;36:2111–8.

96. Glogau R, Blitzer A, Brandt F, et al. Results of a randomized, double-blind, placebo-controlled study to evaluate the efficacy and safety of a botulinum toxin type A topical gel for the treatment of moderate-to-severe lateral canthal lines. J Drugs Dermatol 2012;11(1):38–45.

97. Hsu M, Stevenson FF. Reduction in muscular motility by selective focused cold therapy: a preclinical study. J Neural Transm 2013. [Epub ahead of print].

Filler Placement and the Fat Compartments

Rebecca Fitzgerald, MD*, Ashley G. Rubin, MD

KEYWORDS

- Facial fat compartmentalization • Filler placement • Fat compartments • Facial adipose tissue

KEY POINTS

- Understanding the anatomy and distribution of facial fat and the alterations that occur during the aging process is essential to effectively and precisely achieve facial rejuvenation.
- Over the past several years, through cadaveric dissections and computed tomographic studies, much has been discovered concerning the adipose tissue of the face and how it influences the dynamic process of aging.
- Site-specific augmentation with fillers can now be used to refine facial shape and topography in a more predictable and precise fashion

INTRODUCTION

Our understanding of how the face ages and how to best mitigate these changes, is in a perpetual state of evolution and refinement. Evolving insights into the anatomy of aging are clarifying our understanding of the pathophysiology of aging, the changes in elasticity of the skin, the compartmentalization of facial fat, and the role of bony support and how it changes over time. Seemingly subtle changes over time can have an enormous impact on our perception of a face, making it appear older or younger in an almost imperceptible way. Erasing lines and folds, tightening sagging skin, or restoring young full lips may rejuvenate some faces, but as we are all unfortunately aware, can also look odd and a bit out of perspective on others. Patients new to fillers often bring up fear of this kind of "unnatural" result, causing some to avoid treatments altogether. The restoration of a natural volume distribution is a major goal in facial rejuvenation. Using the evolving knowledge of facial fat anatomy to recognize "what's been lost where" on a case-by-case basis so as to individualize treatment plans may help us to offer the sort of subtle and natural-looking results desired by

many patients ("I don't want to look done, I just don't want to look tired").

The purpose of this article was simply to provide an introduction to some of the recent literature concerning facial fat compartmentalization, along with a few clinical examples that were chosen to illustrate the utility of "site-specific placement" (ie, placing filler in specific fat compartments to obtain specific, predictable, and natural-appearing results). Specific techniques and particular fillers are not addressed here. Additionally, as this article is meant to serve as an introduction to a concept, and not an exhaustive review, more detailed descriptions of this anatomy can be found elsewhere and are referenced in this work.

FACIAL FAT COMPARTMENTS

The discovery that facial fat does not exist as one homogeneous object on the face as traditionally thought, but rather as many dynamic compartments that can be evaluated, augmented, and modified, represents a major breakthrough in our understanding of facial aging.

The central role of volume loss and deflation, rather than ptosis alone, in the aging face has

Division of Dermatology, University of California, Los Angeles (UCLA), 200 Medical Plaza, Suite 450, Los Angeles, CA 90095-6957, USA
* Corresponding author.
E-mail address: fitzmd@earthlink.net

Dermatol Clin 32 (2014) 37–50
http://dx.doi.org/10.1016/j.det.2013.09.007
0733-8635/14/$ – see front matter Published by Elsevier Inc.

been eloquently illustrated by Lambros[1] in a longitudinal photographic analysis of more than 100 patients spanning an average period of 25 years. This invaluable work contributed inspiration to a groundbreaking study done at the University of Texas, Southwestern (UTSW) in 2007, elucidating the compartmentalization of facial fat.[2] Since that time, many subsequent studies from several groups have contributed to this body of knowledge.[3–15] Pessa and Rohrich[16] recently published a textbook presenting findings from more than 1000 dissections encompassing more than 20 years of work that is an excellent resource on this subject.

The landmark studies by Rohrich and Pessa at UTSW utilized fresh cadaveric anatomic dissections with dye staining for visualization of individual compartments. **Fig. 1** shows an image of the superficial fat compartments of the midface from the original study, which revealed the compartmentalization of facial fat in this area. The nasolabial fat compartment is the most medial of the major cheek compartments, followed by the medial and the middle cheek compartments. Subsequent studies revealed that subcutaneous fat, both superficial and deep to the superficial musculoaponeurotic system, is compartmentalized, specifically by fascial extensions that form a framework that provides a "retaining system" for the human face. Implicit in this concept is the

suggestion that the face ages three-dimensionally, with separate compartments changing relative to one another by both position and volume.

The superficial adipose tissue has as its boundaries vascularized membranes arising from superficial fascia, whereas deep fat is compartmentalized by nonvascularized fascial boundaries that most likely represent fusion zones of various fascias.[17]

A working hypothesis of facial fat aging is the concept that folds occur at transition points between thicker and thinner superficial fat compartments; in contrast, loss and/or ptosis of the deep fat compartments leads to changes in contour.[11]

Both may play a role in facial shape, as illustrated by the remaining figures.

UPPER FACE

Fig. 2 shows an image of the lateral temporal cheek fat. The superior and inferior temporal septa (STS and ITS) represent the superior and inferior boundaries, respectively. The temporal fat extends beyond the hairline. This compartment spans the forehead to the cervical region. It is the most lateral of the cheek fat compartments and has an identifiable septal boundary medially called the lateral cheek septum. (The nasolabial

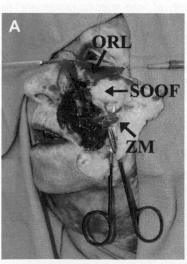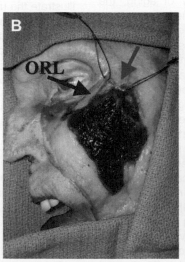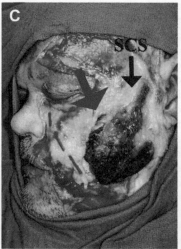

Fig. 1. (*A*) The nasolabial fat compartment is the most medial of the major cheek compartments. Blue dye has stained this region. The orbicularis retaining ligament (ORL) is the superior boundary (*black arrow*). Additional black arrows point to the sub-orbicularis oculi fat (SOOF) and the zygomaticus major muscle (ZM). (*B*) The medial cheek fat compartment lies adjacent to the nasolabial fat. The superior boundary is again the ORL. The red area designates a zone of fixation where this fat compartment intersects with the inferior orbital fat compartment. (*C*) The middle cheek fat compartment is found anterior and superficial to the parotid gland. This compartment is lateral to the medial fat compartment, medial to the lateral temporal-cheek fat, and inferior to the superior cheek septum (SCS). The red arrow designates a zone of fixation between adjacent compartments. (*From* Rohrich RJ, Pessa JE. The fat compartments of the face: anatomy and clinical implications for cosmetic surgery. Plast Reconstr Surg 2007;119:2219–27 [discussion: 2228–31]; with permission.)

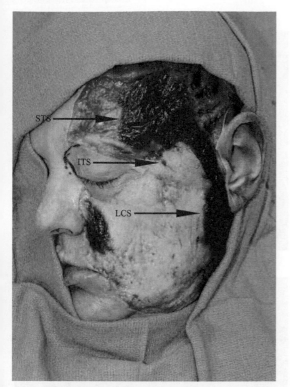

Fig. 2. The lateral temporal-cheek compartment is the most lateral compartment of cheek fat and connects the temporal fat to the cervical subcutaneous fat. The superior and inferior temporal septa (STS and ITS, respectively) represent the superior boundaries, and it has an identifiable septal barrier medially called the lateral cheek septum (LCS). (*From* Rohrich RJ, Pessa JE. The fat compartments of the face: anatomy and clinical implications for cosmetic surgery. Plast Reconstr Surg 2007;119:2219–27 [discussion: 2228–31]; with permission.)

cheek compartment is stained in this image as well. Note the difference in the size of this compartment in this cadaver as opposed to the size of the same compartment in the cadaver pictured in **Fig. 1**.) The clinical photographs in **Figs. 3** and **4** show women who have lost fat in different areas of this compartment with aging. The woman in **Fig. 3**A has lost temporal fat beyond her hairline, changing the shape of her face to a "peanut" shape, which is restored to an oval with volume augmentation in this area. The woman in **Fig. 3**B has lost temporal fat at the superior border, resulting in a somewhat harsh skeletonized appearance that softens with volume augmentation in that area.

The patient in **Fig. 4** has ample temporal volume, but an absence of lateral cheek fat, giving her lateral face a concave (almost "horselike") appearance that is softened as her face is ovalized by treatment in this area. Note that the tragus is

visible in an anterior view in a patient without much lateral cheek fat and is less visible when this area is full (this is often seen in thin patients after facelifting).

Augmenting specific areas has a specific effect and enables the clinician to tailor his or her treatment based on the individual's particular morphology.[18]

The most recent advance in the visualization of these compartments is the use of a novel technique using a thin-slice computed tomographic (CT) scan with an iodinated contrast medium. This method allows for a reproducible three-dimensional (3D) depiction of the compartments that can be used for detailed investigations regarding the shape, size, and volume of the distinct fat compartments.[19,20]

An additional advantage of the use of radiopaque dye with CT is that it allows compartments to be visualized from any plane. Gierloff and colleagues,[19] authors of the first study using this novel technique, studied 12 cadavers divided evenly into younger (59–75) and older (76–104) age groups. They presented evidence that is in concordance with what has been observed in the cadaveric dissection and dye sequestration studies; a schematic from their article depicting the superficial fat compartments of the midface is shown in **Fig. 5**.

In 2007, Rohrich and Pessa[2] determined, via dye injection into cadaveric heads, that there are 3 fat compartments of the forehead. The central compartment is located in the midline and extends inferiorly to the nasal dorsum and laterally to a border that they refer to as the "central temporal septum."

Fig. 6A shows an image of the central forehead compartment in 3D from the Gierloff and colleagues[19] CT study. The forehead is a key area of facial expression. Note in **Fig. 6**B and C that site-specific augmentation of this particular fat pad reduces the perceived look of anger in this patient.

MIDFACE

In 2008, Rohrich and colleagues[8] discovered the deep medial cheek fat compartment that is located just medial to the buccal fat pad and zygomaticus major muscle. This compartment is bounded medially by the pyriform ligament of the nasal base, superiorly by the orbicularis retaining ligament, and lies just deep to the superficial fat compartments. The compartment is distinct from the suborbicularis oculi fat. A potential space exists between the periosteum of the maxilla and the deep medial cheek fat and has been termed "Ristow" space.

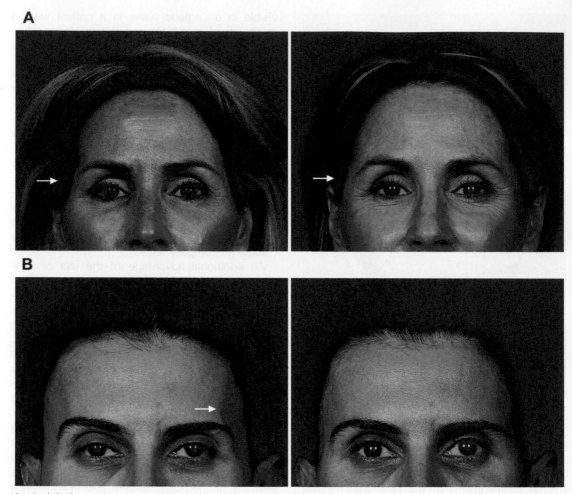

Fig. 3. (*A*) The patient pictured here has lost temporal fat in the area posterior to her hairline. Note that this affects the shape of her face, changing it to a sort of "peanut" shape, which is restored to an oval with volume augmentation in this area. (*B*) The patient here has lost temporal fat at the superior temporal septum (STS) resulting in a somewhat harsh skeletonized appearance, which softens with volume augmentation in that area. (*Courtesy of* Rebecca Fitzgerald, MD, Los Angeles, CA.)

In 2009 an additional study by Rohrich and colleagues[11] showed that the suborbicularis oculi fat (SOOF) is composed of two distinct anatomic compartments. The deep cheek fat is the medial boundary of lower eyelid periorbital submuscular fat. Medial suborbicularis fat is located between deep cheek fat and lateral suborbicularis oculi fat. This lateral compartment extends from the lateral canthus to the lateral orbital thickening.

The CT study by Gierloff and colleagues[19] also provided additional new information concerning deep midfacial fat. Specifically, they noted that the deep medial cheek fat consists of both a medial and lateral compartment, as is seen in the SOOF. These deep midfacial fat compartments are depicted in a schematic from their article in **Fig. 7**. Note the medial extension of the deep medial cheek fat compartment seen around the

pyriform ligament that is not present in the schematic of superficial fat. The investigators of this study also observed radiopaque dye sequestration in a "buccal extension" of the buccal fat pad indicating that this is an independent compartment. This buccal extension of the buccal fat pad is felt by these investigators to play a pivotal role in the support of the compartments above it. Additional new observations made in this study will be discussed later in this section.

Now turn your attention to the patient in **Fig. 8**. Deep midfacial fat is visible clinically. There is no undereye hollowing or nasolabial fold and there is a convex contour to her midface. However, because of a congenital lipodystrophy, there is a striking lack of superficial fat. This is most obvious in her temple and lateral cheek (as well as her periorbital area), but on closer observation the lack of

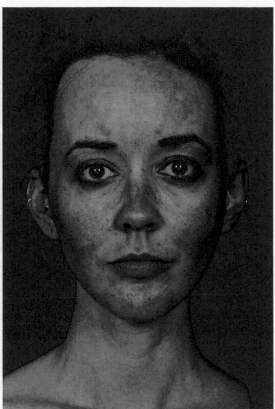

Fig. 4. This patient has ample temporal volume, but an absence of lateral cheek fat, giving her lateral face a concave (almost "horselike") appearance that is softened as her face is ovalized by treatment in this area. Note that the tragus is visible in an anterior view in a patient without much lateral cheek fat and is less visible when this area is full (this is often seen in thin patients after facelifting). (*Courtesy of* Rebecca Fitzgerald, MD, Los Angeles, CA.)

superficial fat in her midface is causing a good deal of shadowing. This shadowing corrects with treatment in the areas of the superficial medial and middle cheek fat compartments.

Fig. 9 is a three-dimensional image of the medial part of the deep medial cheek compartment showing fat extending under the nasolabial fold, as well as up to the inferior border of the orbital rim. It easy to appreciate what the clinical effects of a treatment in this specific area might accomplish. The dotted red line represents the nasolabial fold. The lateral part of the deep medial cheek

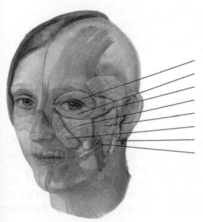

Superior orbital fat
Inferior orbital fat
Lateral orbital fat
Medial cheek fat
Middle cheek fat
Nasolabial fat
Lateral temporal-cheek fat
Buccal extension of the buccal fat

Fig. 5. Stylistic drawing of the anatomic relationships of the facial fat compartments. The midfacial fat is arranged in 2 and paranasally in 3 independent anatomic layers. The superficial layer (*yellow*) is composed of the nasolabial fat, the medial cheek fat, the middle cheek fat, the lateral temporal cheek compartment, and 3 orbital compartments. (*From* Gierloff M, Stöhring C, Buder T, et al. Aging changes of the midfacial fat compartments: a computed tomographic study. Plast Reconstr Surg 2012;129(1):263–73; with permission.)

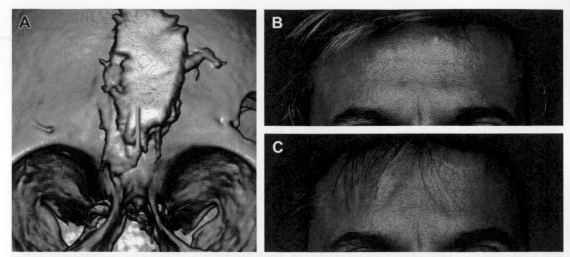

Fig. 6. (A) CT image of the subcutaneous central forehead compartment. The yellow line indicates the position of the glabellar fold that is located superficially to the inferior portion of the compartment. (B, C) Note that site-specific augmentation of this particular fat pad reduces the perceived look of anger in this patient. ([A] *From* Gierloff M, Stöhring C, Buder T, et al. The subcutaneous fat compartments in relation to aesthetically important facial folds and rhytides. J Plast Reconstr Aesthet Surg 2012;65(10):1292–7, with permission; and [B, C] *Courtesy of* Rebecca Fitzgerald, MD, Los Angeles, CA.)

compartment is not shown. An elevation and effacement of the nasolabial fold can be achieved by augmentation of the deep medial cheek fat (medial part) and augmentation of the deepest fat compartment in the paranasal region ("Ristow" space), which both extend further medially than the overlying nasolabial fold. In contrast, because of the topography, the lateral part of the deep medial cheek fat is responsible for the anterior cheek projection. This is well illustrated by the

image in **Fig. 10**, where the deep medial cheek compartment has been filled with saline in a cadaver. Note the effacement of the nasolabial fold and undereye hollowing as well as the projection and shape of the cheek. Note that the black arrow shows how the skin stretches as this area is filled.

Look now at **Fig. 11** for clinical examples of treatment in the same area. Again, treatment of this one area leads to effacement of the nasolabial

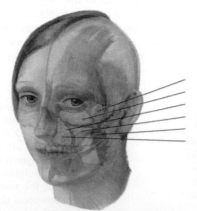

Sub–orbicularis oculi fat (lateral part)
Sub–orbicularis oculi fat (medial part)
Deep medial cheek fat (medial part)
Deep medial cheek fat (lateral part)
Buccal extension of the buccal fat
Ristow's space

Fig. 7. Stylistic drawing of the anatomic relationships of deep midfacial fat compartments. It is composed of the suborbicularis oculi fat (medial and lateral parts) and the deep medial cheek fat (medial and lateral parts). Three layers of distinct fat compartments are found laterally to the pyriform aperture, where a deep compartment (*blue*) is located posterior to the medial part of the deep medial cheek fat. The buccal extension of the buccal fat pad extends from the paramaxillary space to the subcutaneous plane. (*From* Gierloff M, Stöhring C, Buder T, et al. Aging changes of the midfacial fat compartments: a computed tomographic study. Plast Reconstr Surg 2012;129(1):263–73; with permission.)

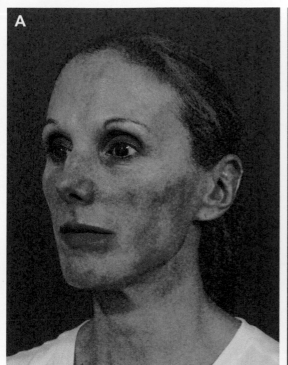
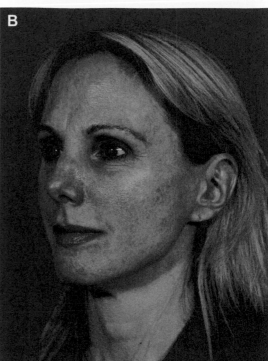

Fig. 8. (A) Deep midfacial fat is visible clinically. There is no undereye hollowing or nasolabial fold and there is a convex contour to her midface. However, due to a congenital lipodystrophy, there is a striking lack of superficial fat. This is most obvious in her temple and lateral cheek (as well as her periorbital area), but on closer observation the lack of superficial fat in her midface is causing a good deal of shadowing. (B) This shadowing corrects with treatment in the areas of the superficial medial and middle cheek fat compartments. (*Courtesy of* Rebecca Fitzgerald, MD, Los Angeles, CA.)

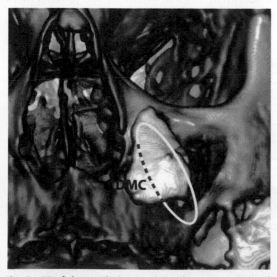

Fig. 9. CT of the medial part of the deep medial cheek fat (DMC). The yellow line indicates the position of the overlying nasolabial fat compartment. The red dashed line indicates the course of the nasolabial crease. (*From* Gierloff M, Stöhring C, Buder T, et al. The subcutaneous fat compartments in relation to aesthetically important facial folds and rhytides. J Plast Reconstr Aesthet Surg 2012;65(10):1292–7; with permission.)

fold and improvement in undereye hollowing. Obviously, the older patient (see **Fig. 11**A) with more volume loss required more product for this result than the younger patient (see **Fig. 11**B) with less volume loss. Note that the area of the lateral SOOF in both of these patients had volume before this treatment and therefore blends in well with the newly treated area. In the cadaver in the previous image, volume restoration of the deep medial cheek fat makes the lack of volume in his lateral SOOF even more obvious. This area clearly did not fill with the treatment shown, because it is a separate fat compartment not accessed by the treatment. This anatomy has enormous clinical relevance in facial filling, as it allows specific areas to be targeted for specific effects. Lack of volume in the lateral SOOF truncates the cheek. Treatment in the area of the lateral SOOF augments the prominence of the cheek.[16]

This effect is well illustrated by the clinical image seen in **Fig. 12**. At first glance, the issue seems to be a prominent nasolabial fold, but knowledge of the specific fat compartments facilitates recognition of the relatively empty medial and lateral SOOF compartments. Treatment in these fat pads

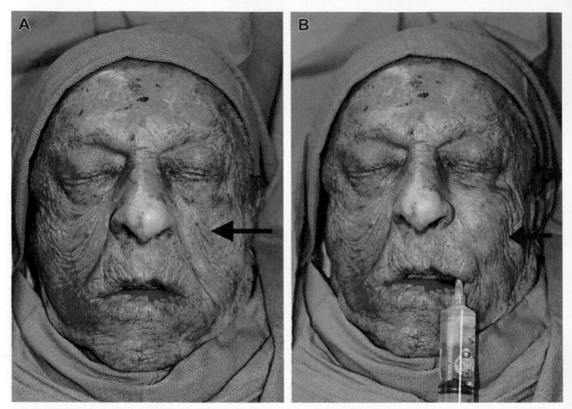

Fig. 10. Photograph of a deflated midface (*A*). (*B*) Saline injected specifically into the deep medial cheek fat restores anterior projection, diminishes the nasolabial fold, and effaces the nasojugal trough. Note that the cheek has a natural appearance. Recognize that this is because the fascial boundaries of the deep medial cheek compartment determine and define its shape. This means that filler placed specifically into this fat compartment will reflect this shape and have a natural appearance. (*From* Rohrich RJ, Pessa JE, Ristow BR. The youthful cheek and the deep medial fat compartment. Plast Reconstr Surg 2008;121:2107–12; with permission.)

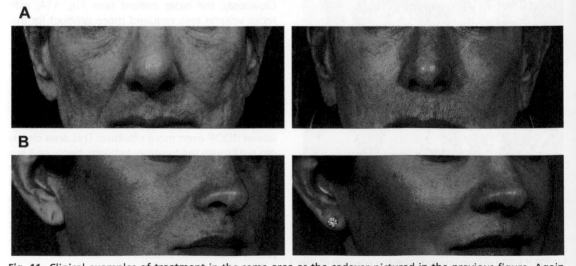

Fig. 11. Clinical examples of treatment in the same area as the cadaver pictured in the previous figure. Again, treatment of this one area leads to effacement of the nasolabial fold and improvement in undereye hollowing. Obviously, the older patient (*A*) with more volume loss required more product for this result than the younger patient (*B*) with less volume loss. Note that the area of the lateral SOOF in both of these patients had volume before this treatment and therefore blends in well with the newly treated area. In the cadaver in the previous image, volume restoration of the deep medial cheek fat makes the lack of volume in his lateral SOOF even more obvious. (*Courtesy of* Rebecca Fitzgerald, MD, Los Angeles, CA.)

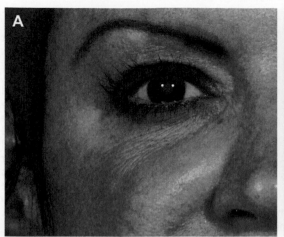
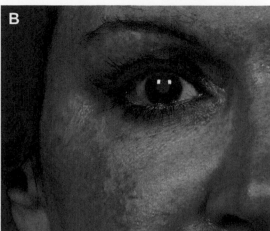

Fig. 12. (A) At first glance, the patient's issue seems to be a prominent nasolabial fold, but knowledge of the specific fat compartments facilitates recognition of the relatively empty medial and lateral SOOF compartments. (B) Treatment in these fat pads achieves a natural-appearing correction. This patient was also treated with neuromodulators and filler in the brow. (*Courtesy of* Rebecca Fitzgerald, MD, Los Angeles, CA.)

achieve a natural-appearing correction. This patient was also treated with neuromodulators and filler in the brow.

The patient in **Fig. 13** was treated in the deep medial cheek fat as well as in the medial and lateral SOOF. The volumization of the lateral SOOF can be most appreciated on the right side of her face in this three-quarter view. This patient was treated with neuromodulators and filler in the brow fat as well.

These specific areas of treatment are well illustrated in the 3-D CT image in **Fig. 14**, which shows both the medial aspect of the deep medial cheek fat

on the right as well as the medial and lateral SOOF on the left. This image also illustrates 2 important new observations made possible by the use of the 3D technique by Gierloff and colleagues.[19] They studied 12 cadavers divided evenly into a younger (59–75) and an older (76–104) age group. They observed (1) an inferior migration or "sagging" of the midfacial fat compartments and (2) an inferior volume shift within the compartments in the older versus younger group.

For evaluation of the "sagging" of the compartments, the distance between the cephalad border and the infraorbital rim was determined. For

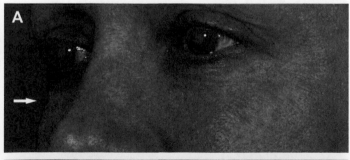
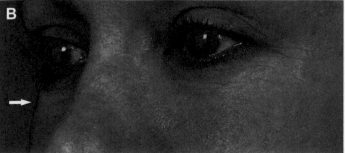

Fig. 13. (A) Prior to treatment. (B) This patient was treated in the deep medial cheek fat as well as in the medial and lateral SOOF. The volumization of the lateral SOOF can be most appreciated on the right side of her face in this three-quarter view. This patient was treated with neuromodulators and filler in the brow fat as well. (*Courtesy of* Rebecca Fitzgerald, MD, Los Angeles, CA.)

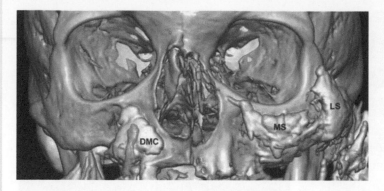

Fig. 14. The deep midfacial fat compartments. The deep medial cheek fat is composed of a medial part (DMC) and a lateral part (not shown). The medial part extends medially almost to the lateral incisor tooth. Augmentation of the deep medial cheek fat will consequently elevate and efface the nasolabial fold. The suborbicularis oculi fat is composed of a medial part (MS) and a lateral part (LS). With aging, an inferior migration of these compartments occurs, as well as an inferior volume shift within the compartments. (*From* Gierloff M, Stöhring C, Buder T, et al. Aging changes of the midfacial fat compartments: a computed tomographic study. Plast Reconstr Surg 2012;129(1):263–73; with permission.)

evaluation of the volume distribution within a specific compartment, the sagittal diameter of the upper, middle, and lower thirds of each compartment was determined. Representation of both of these changes can be appreciated in this image.

The investigators noted that these observations are consistent with some of the changes we see with aging. For instance, volume loss of the cephalad part of the nasolabial and medial cheek fat would consequently worsen the appearance of the tear trough deformity, the nasojugal fold, and the palpebromalar groove. A volume increase

of the inferior part of the nasolabial fat would lead to a pronounced nasolabial fold and a pronounced superior jowl. Also, inferior migration of the fat compartments could contribute to the crescent-shaped hollow below the lower edge of the orbicularis oculi muscle and the deepening of the nasojugal fold seen with aging.[19]

LOWER FACE

Finally, let's take a look at the perioral area of the lower face. **Fig. 15** shows a cadaveric dissection

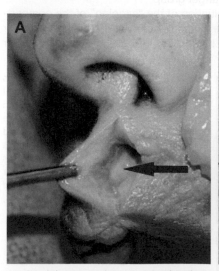
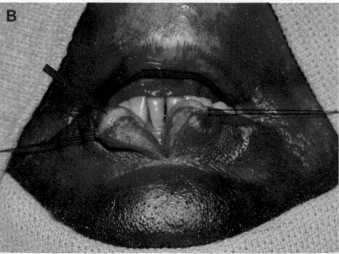

Fig. 15. (A) Just as there is suborbicularis fat around the eye, there is suborbicularis fat of the perioral region. Histologic examination confirms the macroscopic finding that the orbicularis insertion defines the wet-dry border of the lip. Vertical sectioning of the upper lip reveals fat deep to the orbicularis oris muscle (*arrow*) and superficial to the buccal mucosa. (B) Vertical sectioning of the lower lip again shows deep submuscular fat (*arrow*). Of particular note, this specimen's lower lip showed anterior projection and eversion similar to that seen in a much younger individual. The clinical impression from this research is that the volume of deep lip fat contributes significantly to the appearance of the youthful lip. ([B] *From* Rohrich RJ, Pessa JE, Ristow BR. The youthful cheek and the deep medial fat compartment. Plast Reconstr Surg 2008;121:2107–12; and Rohrich R, Pessa J. The anatomy and clinical implications of perioral submuscular fat. Plast Reconstr Surg 2009:124(1):266–71; with permission.)

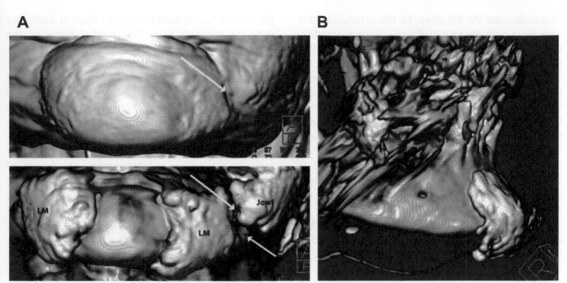

Fig. 16. (A) Images of a volume-rendered 3D spiral CT of the lower face demonstrating the surface of the skin (above) and the anterior part of the mandible with the labiomandibular fat compartments (LM) and the left inferior jowl fat (below). The yellow arrows indicate the position of the labiomandibular fold. The white arrow indicates the position of the mandibular retaining ligament. (B) Images of a volume-rendered 3D spiral CT of the chin demonstrating the submentalis fat. Note that this compartment deso not lie immediately adjacent to the mentolabial sulcus. (From Gierloff M, Stöhring C, Buder T, et al. The subcutaneous fat compartments in relation to aesthetically important facial folds and rhytides. J Plast Reconstr Aesthet Surg 2012;65(10):1292–7; with permission.)

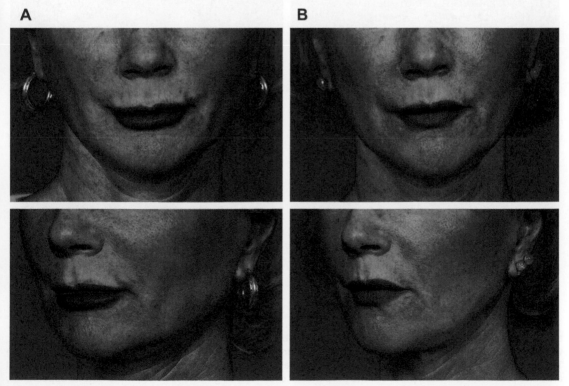

Fig. 17. (A) Following previous injection the patient's lips appeared unnatural. (B) Removing suboptimally placed filler in the vermillion border (with hyaluronidase) followed by placement of filler in a submuscular location in the mucosal and cutaneous portion of the patient's upper and lower lip as well as in her lateral and anterior chin provide more support for her lips and a more natural appearing result. (Courtesy of Rebecca Fitzgerald, MD, Los Angeles, CA.)

that illustrates the fat deep to the orbicularis oris muscle in both the mucosal and cutaneous portion of the upper and lower lips. It is thought that this fat may help facilitate eversion in a young lip, whereas the lack of this support may contribute to the inversion seen in an older lip.[10] **Fig. 16** shows images of a volume-rendered 3-D spiral CT of the lower face demonstrating the surface of the skin (above) and the anterior part of the mandible, with the labiomandibular fat compartments and the left inferior jowl fat (below). The yellow arrows indicate the position of the labiomandibular fold. The white arrow indicates the position of the mandibular retaining ligament.

One layer of fat was identified in the region of the labiomandibular fold (marionette line). The labiomandibular crease lies between the labiomandibular fat compartment (LM) and the jowl fat, as indicated by the yellow line. The lateral edge of the LM appeared to be thinner in cadavers with a prominent labiomandibular fold than in cadavers with no obvious fold. The medial edge of the depressor anguli oris muscle follows the course of the crease.

Knowledge of this anatomy enables correction of the suboptimal placement of lip filler seen in the patient shown in **Fig. 17**. Fear of this unnatural "duck" lip is probably one of the most common patient concerns we hear regarding lip augmentation. Removing the filler in the vermillion border (with hyaluronidase), followed by placement of filler in a submuscular location in the mucosal and cutaneous portion of her upper and lower lip as well as in her lateral and anterior chin provide more support for her lips and a more natural-appearing result.

In the final clinical example shown in **Fig. 18**, we see a patient who has been treated suboptimally in the tear trough area with hyaluronic acid. This resulted in an unnatural convexity to her infraorbital

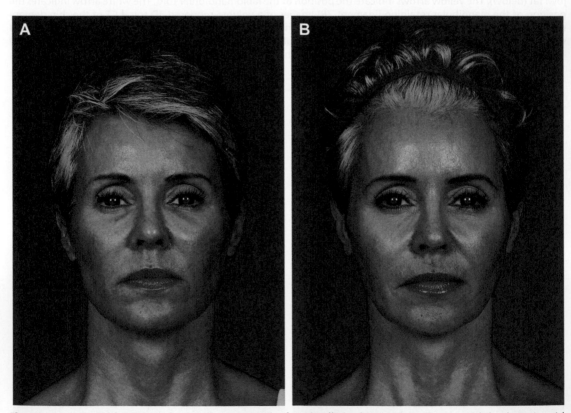

Fig. 18. A 51-year-old patient who has been treated suboptimally in the tear trough area with hyaluronic acid, which gives an unnatural convexity to her infraorbital area as well as a bluish reflection (referred to as both the Tyndall effect and Raleigh scattering). Hyaluronidase was used to remove the hyaluronic acid in the infraorbital area and product was instead placed in the deep medial cheek fat. To give her a softer, more natural appearance, she also received treatment in the lateral temporal-cheek fat pad, both behind the hairline and along the superior and inferior temporal septa, as shown in **Fig. 3**. She was also treated in the lateral cheek fat, as shown in **Fig. 4**, as well as in the medial and lateral SOOF. Finally, to correct the mild shadowing noted in her midface, the superficial medial and middle cheek fats were also treated, as depicted in **Fig. 8**. (*Courtesy of* Rebecca Fitzgerald, MD, Los Angeles, CA.)

area as well as a bluish reflection referred to as both the Tyndall effect and Raleigh scattering. Hyaluronidase was used to remove the hyaluronic acid in the infraorbital area and product was instead placed in the deep medial cheek fat.

To give her a softer, more natural appearance, she also received treatment in the lateral temporal-cheek fat pad, both behind the hairline and along the superior and inferior temporal septa, as previously shown in **Fig. 3**. She was also treated in the lateral cheek fat as previously shown in **Fig. 4**, as well as in the medial and lateral SOOF. Finally, to correct the mild shadowing noted in her midface, the superficial medial and middle cheek fats were also treated, as previously depicted in **Fig. 8**.

SUMMARY

To summarize, the superficial fat is composed of the nasolabial, medial cheek, middle cheek, and lateral temporal cheek compartments, the three superficial periorbital compartments (as seen in the schematic in **Fig. 5**), as well as the three forehead compartments. The deep adipose layer is composed of the suborbicularis fat and the deep medial cheek fat, each with a medial and lateral compartment (as seen in the schematic in **Fig. 7**). Three layers of distinct fat compartments are found just lateral to the pyriform aperture, where a compartment termed "Ristow" space is located posterior to the medial part of the deep medial cheek fat. These findings are in concordance in all studies to date.

The most recent advance is a new method using contrast CT, which allows a reproducible 3-D depiction of the compartments that can be used for detailed investigations regarding the shape, size, and volume of the distinct fat compartments. This technique also allows compartments to be visualized from any plane.

The first study using this method found that a "buccal extension" of the buccal fat exists as an independent fat compartment and may play a pivotal role in the aging face. Two other significant observations made in this study were (1) an inferior migration of the midfacial fat compartments and (2) an inferior volume shift within the compartments occurs during aging.

The information garnered from both cadaveric dissections and CT studies have important aesthetic clinical implications. Site-specific augmentation with fillers (or fat) can now be used to refine facial shape and topography in a more predictable and precise fashion. The purpose of this article has been simply to provide a few clinical examples to illustrate this concept. There is still

much to be learned about the underlying anatomy of facial adipose tissue and the changes that occur through the aging process, as well as how to best apply this knowledge clinically. The ability to determine the physiologic size and shape of each facial fat compartment, including its age-dependent changes, would allow us to redistribute the fat of each compartment in a physiologic way and mimic the facial fat distribution in youth. This would not only lead to a more natural volume distribution, but also enable a smaller consumption of fat or filler.

Of course, a major limitation that is present in all of the studies presented is the lack of longitudinality. Eventually, as longitudinal studies are undertaken, we will know more regarding the dynamic changes that occur within and between each fat compartment with aging.

We all recognize that optimal, predictable, and reproducible patient outcomes are best facilitated by carefully predicting (patient selection), planning (facial analysis and mapping), and performing (proper preparation and injection of product) treatments in an informed manner. It is our hope that the information provided here will help to facilitate this goal. We look forward to further developments in this interesting and fascinating field.

REFERENCES

1. Lambros V. Observations on periorbital and midfacial aging. Plast Reconstr Surg 2007;120:1367–76.
2. Rohrich RJ, Pessa JE. The fat compartments of the face: Anatomy and clinical implications for cosmetic surgery. Plast Reconstr Surg 2007;119: 2219–27 [discussion: 2228–31].
3. Hwang SH, Hwang K, Jin S, et al. Location and nature of retro-orbicularis oculus fat and sub–orbicularis oculi fat. J Craniofac Surg 2007;18:387–90.
4. Ghavami A, Pessa J, Janis J, et al. The orbicularis retaining ligament of the medial orbit: closing the circle. Plast Reconstr Surg 2008;121(3):994–1001.
5. Reece EM, Pessa JE, Rohrich RJ. The mandibular septum: anatomical observations of the jowls in aging. Implications for facial rejuvenation. Plast Reconstr Surg 2008;121:1414–20.
6. Garcia de Mitchell CA, Pessa JE, Schaverien MV, et al. The philtrum: anatomical observations from a new perspective. Plast Reconstr Surg 2008;122: 1756–60.
7. Rohrich RJ, Pessa JE. The retaining system of the face: histologic evaluation of the septal boundaries of the subcutaneous fat compartments. Plast Reconstr Surg 2008;121:1804–9.
8. Rohrich RJ, Pessa JE, Ristow BR. The youthful cheek and the deep medial fat compartment. Plast Reconstr Surg 2008;121:2107–12.

9. Rohrich RJ, Ahmad J, Hamawy AH, et al. Is the intra-orbital fat extraorbital? Results of cross-sectional anatomy of the lower eyelid fat pads. Aesthet Surg J 2009;29:189–93.

10. Rohrich R, Pessa J. The anatomy and clinical implications of perioral submuscular fat. Plast Reconstr Surg 2009;124(1):266–71.

11. Rohrich RJ, Arbique GM, Wong C, et al. The anatomy of sub–orbicularis oculi fat: implications for periorbital rejuvenation. Plast Reconstr Surg 2009; 124:946–51.

12. Schaverien MV, Pessa JE, Rohrich RJ. Vascularized membranes determine the anatomical boundaries of the subcutaneous fat compartments. Plast Reconstr Surg 2009;123:695–700.

13. Pilsl U, Anderhuber F. The chin and adjacent fat compartments. Dermatol Surg 2010;36:214–8.

14. Pilsl U, Anderhuber F. The septum subcutaneum parotideomassetericum. Dermatol Surg 2010;36: 2005–8.

15. Rohrich R, Taylor N, Ahmad J, et al. Great auricular nerve injury, the "subauricular band" phenomenon, and the periauricular adipose compartments. Plast Reconstr Surg 2011;127(2):835–43.

16. Pessa JE, Rohrich RJ. Facial topography. Clinical anatomy of the face. St Louis (MO): Quality Medical Publishing, Inc; 2012.

17. Rohrich R, Pessa J. Discussion: aging changes of the midfacial fat compartments: a computed tomographic study. Plast Reconstr Surg 2012;129(1):274–5.

18. Sandoval SE, Cox JA, Koshy JC, et al. Facial fat compartments: a guide to filler placement. Semin Plast Surg 2009;23(4):283–7.

19. Gierloff M, Stöhring C, Buder T, et al. Aging changes of the midfacial fat compartments: a computed tomographic study. Plast Reconstr Surg 2012;129(1):263–73.

20. Gierloff M, Stöhring C, Buder T, et al. The subcutaneous fat compartments in relation to aesthetically important facial folds and rhytides. J Plast Reconstr Aesthet Surg 2012;65(10):1292–7.

A Modern Approach to the Treatment of Cellulite

Anthony M. Rossi, MD[a,b], Bruce E. Katz, MD[b,c],*

KEYWORDS

- Cellulite • Laser lipolysis • Skin laxity • Nd: YAG laser for cellulite

KEY POINTS

- Cellulite is a well-documented condition and, although many treatment options have been purported, few have lasting clinical results.
- The use of laser and light-based devices, in both a noninvasive and a minimally invasive fashion, has augmented the understanding and approach to the treatment of cellulite.
- Understanding the structural components that underpin cellulite anatomy allows for a more specific targeting approach.

INTRODUCTION

Cellulite is a topographic alteration of the skin and subcutaneous adipose that has been reported as early as 150 years ago but yet still affects patients today. It is quite prevalent, almost ubiquitous in postpubertal women and can be thought of as a female secondary sex characteristic.[1] Cellulite formation has a complex pathophysiology that includes expansion of subcutaneous fat, fibrotic dermal septae, as well as dermal laxity and atrophy. Many factors are also thought to influence the formation of cellulite; a genetic predisposition, along with hormonal influences, structural adipose differences, and inflammation may all contribute. It is thought that in cellulite the adipose cells are arranged in chambers surrounded by bands of connective tissue called septae, which span to connect muscle to the inferior portion of the dermis. The adipose cells that are encased within the perimeters of this area expand with water absorption, thereby stretching the connective tissue.

This connective tissue can contract and thicken, holding the skin at a nonflexible length, while the surrounding tissue continues to expand with weight, or water gain. This expansion results in skin dimpling and an orange peel appearance, mainly in the pelvis, thighs, and abdominal areas.[2] Many devices and treatments have focused on these purported structural alterations as targets for therapy, some with better results than others. Even with many technological and pharmacologic advances, cellulite has been extremely recalcitrant to a wide array of treatments.

CELLULITE ANATOMY AND GRADING

The topographic appearance of cellulite is multifactorial in nature. The overall contour deformity is that of skin depression admixed with lax inelastic epidermis. The area of cellulite can comprise isolated depressions or a cluster of such that leads to an overall rippled appearance. The depressed areas can be either ovoid or linear in

Anthony M. Rossi MD has nothing to disclose.
Bruce E. Katz, MD has the following disclosures: Alma, Clinical Advisory Board; Life Biosciences, Consultant; Merz Pharmaceuticals, Clinical Advisory Board; El-En Engineering, Consultant; Cynosure, Stockholder; Valeant Pharm, Clinical Advisory Board; Allergan, Clinical Advisory Board.
a Memorial Sloan Kettering Cancer Center, Weill Cornell Medical College, 1275 York Avenue, New York, NY 10065, USA; b Juva Skin & Laser Center, 60 East 56 Street, New York, NY 10022, USA; c Mt. Sinai School of Medicine, Cosmetic Surgery & Laser Clinic, Mt. Sinai Medical Center, One Gustave L. Levy Place, New York, NY 10029-6574, USA
* Corresponding author. Juva Skin and Laser Center, 60 East 56 Street, New York, NY 10022.
E-mail address: brukatz@gmail.com

Dermatol Clin 32 (2014) 51–59
http://dx.doi.org/10.1016/j.det.2013.09.005

derm.theclinics.com

shape. Ovoid areas of cellulite tend to be more prominent on the buttocks or posterior thigh regions. Cellulite can be broken down into 3 main structural components: (1) adipocytes and collections of fat cells that are arranged in clusters surrounded by bands of connective tissue; (2) these connective tissue septae, which connect underlying muscle to the subdermal layer; (3) cells held within the perimeters of this area expand and stretch the connective tissue. Eventually this connective tissue contracts and sclerosis holds the skin at a nonflexible length, while the surrounding tissue continues to expand with weight, or water gain. Nurnberger and Muller[3] described an anatomic hypothesis of cellulite based on gender-related differences in the structural characteristics of dermal architecture. They reported that dermal septae of affected women are thinner and more radially oriented than those of unaffected men; this facilitates herniation of adipose tissue into the dermis.

GRADING

There are multiple scales of cellulite grading based on the clinical severity. Nurnberger and Muller described a scale of 3 grades:

- Grade I: Skin is smooth when standing.

- Grade II, mild, moderate, severe: Grade II is defined as orange peel or mattress appearance when standing.
- Grade III, mild, moderate, severe: Grade III is defined as grade II cellulite plus raised and depressed areas and nodules when standing (**Fig. 1**).

Curri also described a cellulite grading scale, ranging from grade 0 (absence of cellulite) to grade III cellulite (skin dimpling on standing as well as in supine position and can be exacerbated by skin pinching). It is important to grade the severity of cellulite properly to gauge which treatment would be most effective.

Before any procedure, the physician should take a thorough medical history and physical examination of the area (**Box 1**). It is important to note any bleeding problems or infections in the past. The time course when the patient first noted the cellulitic areas should be ascertained along with a history of any previous surgical or noninvasive procedures. Any trauma of the area should be ascertained. Also any lymphatic or vascular insufficiency or surgery of the area should be assessed. For any nonsurgical or surgical procedures, a medication and allergy history should be taken, highlighting any medications that interact with the cytochrome P450 enzymes.

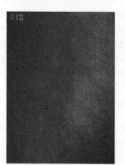 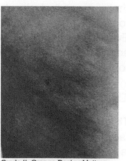  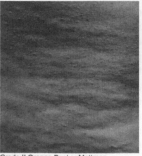

Grade I - Skin is smooth when standing | Grade II Orange Peel or Mattress appearance when standing - MILD | Grade II Orange Peel or Mattress appearance when standing - MODERATE | Grade II Orange Peel or Mattress appearance when standing - SEVERE

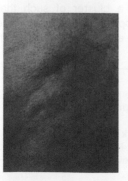 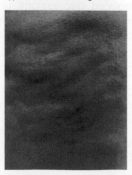 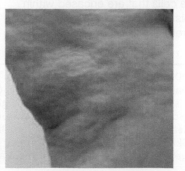

Grade III - Grade II cellulite plus raised and depressed areas and nodules when standing - MILD | Grade III - Grade II cellulite plus raised and depressed areas and nodules when standing - MODERATE | Grade III - Grade II cellulite plus raised and depressed areas and nodules when standing - SEVERE

Fig. 1. Modified Muller Nuremberger scale showing different grades of cellulite.

The physical examination should be done with the patient standing to account for the force of gravity and any asymmetry should be meticulously noted. When examining the area of cellulite, the pinch test can be used, or the patient can contract the muscles in the area, to accentuate the dimpling of the cellulite. The pinch test is done by pinching the area of interest between the thumb and index finger. Tangential lighting can also aid in the visualization of cellulite because this allows for more inspection of contour irregularities. Baseline body weight and body mass index should be recorded. Also circumferential measurements of the area being evaluated (bilateral thighs, hips, or waist) may be taken. Even depths of individual cellulite depressions can be measured at baseline to compare after treatment.

BASELINE PHOTOGRAPHY

Appropriate imaging pretreatment is important to gauge any improvement after treatment. Cellulite photography and imaging can be quite altered by lighting and shadowing due to the undulating and rippling topographic nature of the condition. Therefore proper lighting and positioning of the patient is key. Overhead or tangential illumination of the areas should be used to visualize the surface area better. Photographs should be taken with the patient standing and muscles relaxed. A total body photograph as well as multiple close-up photos of the individual areas should be taken. These photographs can then be used to have an open and frank discussion with the patient about the severity and grading of the cellulite, as well as realistic outcomes that are possible. Another option for imaging is a 3D imaging system, such as the Vectra system (Canfield Scientific, Fairfield, NJ, USA). This technology is passive stereo photogrammetry that uses stereo-paired cameras to map out surface features. Passive stereo photogrammetry is immune to subject movement and also negates the effects of ambient room lightening. The imaging software also calculates the surface height and volume change within the treatment area **(Fig. 2)**.

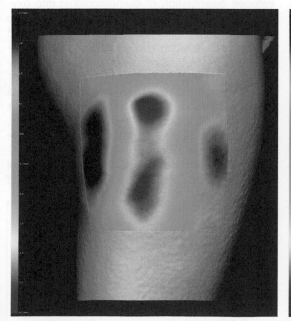

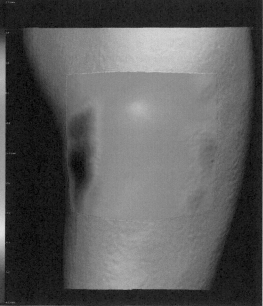

Baseline-red area indicates depression of skin   6 Months post op showing elevation of depressed area

Fig. 2. 3D imaging analysis methodology.

PHARMACOLOGIC TREATMENT OPTIONS

The treatment armamentarium targeted toward cellulite includes weight loss, topical pharmacologic agents, and physical mechanisms. The main pharmacologic treatment options include methylxanthines (caffeine, aminophylline, and theophylline) and retinol.

Methylxanthines

Aminophylline is a compound formed from the combination of ethylene diamine in anhydrous alcohol and theophylline. It acts as an inhibitor of phosphodiesterase, which breaks down cyclic adenosine monophosphate. Its purported mechanism in cellulite treatment is through the "metabolism" of fat and cellulite by stimulating $\alpha\beta2$-adipocyte receptors, which can release adipose stores.

In one study 12 patients applied 5 mL of 2% aminophylline solution on the thigh and buttocks area twice a day. Patients were assessed 1 hour after first application and then subsequently at 3 weeks, 6 weeks, and 3 months. Although photographs showed varying degrees of improvement, 8 subjects demonstrated thinning of the subcutaneous layer on ultrasound taken at 3 months compared with baseline. However, Collis and colleagues[4] evaluated the effectiveness of topical aminophylline gel in combination with 10% glycolic acid and reported no statistically significant improvement.

Retinoids

The idea that cellulite is partly composed of a weakened dermis and herniating fat protuberance leads to the thought that retinoids could treat such weakened dermis and herniating fat protuberance. Retinoid compounds are known to increase dermal collagen fibers and this is speculated to improve cellulite by preventing further herniation of fat. Kligman and colleagues[5] conducted a study of 19 women, who were given 0.3% retinol cream over a period of 6 months twice a day and showed improvement in the side treated with retinol compared with placebo. The observer noted improvement in 12 of the 19 subjects, rating 5 subjects as having good improvement and 7 subjects as having fair improvement. Laser Doppler velocimetry was also used and showed an increase in blood flow in the area treated with the retinoid compound as opposed to the placebo-treated thigh. Ultrasound measured an increase in dermal thickness from 1.44 mm to 1.60 mm, which is statistically significant compared with placebo.

NONPHARMACOLOGIC TREATMENT OPTIONS

A myriad of noninvasive devices has been produced for the treatment of cellulite, all with varying results (Box 2). Some combine suction and massage, whereas others use laser and light sources to target adipose cells. Anderson and colleagues[6] purported that the 1210-nm and 1720-nm wavelengths are selectively absorbed by adipose cells and from this concluded that wavelengths in the infrared spectrum can be used for selective photothermolysis of fat. Although laser platforms in combination with liposuction have been used for lipolysis, there have also been laser-assisted devices designed for cellulite treatment. Other devices have used radiofrequency or ultrasound technology to heat up and destroy the structural components that make up cellulite pathophysiology. Drawbacks to noninvasive modalities include the need for multiple sessions and maintenance treatment.

Both the VelaSmooth and VelaShape (Syneron Medical Ltd, Yokneam Illit, Israel) use radiofrequency energy as well as infrared light wavelengths to treat cellulite noninvasively. The infrared light spectrum ranges from 680 to 1500 nm and can possibly penetrate up to 5 mm below the skin.[7]

Velasmooth is US Food and Drug Administration (FDA) –approved and combines infrared light, bipolar radiofrequency, suction, and massage. The radiofrequency is postulated to target the connective tissue septa and fat whereas the infrared light induces dissociation of oxyhemoglobin into oxygen and hemoglobin, which allows the oxygen to be more readily available for fat metabolism and coupled with suction and massage, improves circulation and stretches connective tissue surrounding adipose collections.[8]

Alster and colleagues[9] studied 20 participants who were treated with 8 sessions each (twice a week for 1 month) on the thigh and buttock areas. They were graded for improvement on a quartile percentage scale (grade 0–4). Eighteen of 20 patients saw an improvement in the appearance of their cellulite 1 month after the completion of

---

Box 2
Noninvasive treatment options

Suction and massage	Endermologie
Radiofrequency (RF) and infrared	Velasmooth, Velashape
Bipolar and unipolar RF	Accent
Monopolar RF	Exilis
Ultrasound	Ultrashape
Laser/light therapies	SmoothShapes, TriActive

treatment, with the average graded score being 1.82. However, at follow-up appointments, the graded score decreased to 1.4 at 3 months and to about 1.1 at 6 months. This decrease in graded score highlights the need for re-treatment to maintain results. In a study conducted by Sadick and Magro[10] in which biopsy specimens were taken, no changes were seen on biopsy.

The Alma Accent Radiofrequency system is FDA-approved for the treatment of rhytides and wrinkles that has been used to treat cellulite (not FDA approved). It uses bipolar and unipolar radiofrequencies. The RF waves are thought to excite electrons, causing rotation of water molecules in the tissue, which then generates energy. This generated heat energy is thought to cause collagen contraction and collagen denaturation.

del Pino and colleagues[11] conducted a study of the unipolar RF mode Accent, in which 26 women received 2 treatment sessions on the buttocks and thighs. Ultrasound measurements were taken to measure the thickness difference between the Camper's fascia and deep dermis and from the deeper dermis to the muscle. Fifteen patients showed a 20% contraction of volume. Ultrasound showed an increase of fibrous tissue and in thickness of these fibers, presumed to be affecting the collagen. Six months after the completion of the study, the patients not lost to follow-up still showed the improved body contouring effects.

Another study of 30 patients in which magnetic resonance imaging measurements and histologic samples were taken showed posttreatment dermal fibrosis histologically but no changes on magnetic resonance imaging. It was concluded that the dermal fibrosis leads to the changes seen clinically.[12]

Ultrashape is not FDA-approved for cellulite treatment. This technology uses ultrasound via a transducer. The transducer contains multiple transducers including a therapeutic focused transducer connected to a power unit for ultrasound energy delivery to selected depths and is thought to produce adipose cell lysis without excessive damage to underlying vasculature, nerves bundles, lymphatics, or connective tissue/musculature. Its role in cellulite treatment has not been extensively studied.

The TriActive (Cynosure, Westford, MA, USA) platform used 3 components to treat cellulite specifically: contact cooling, massage, and a diode laser. Schindl and colleagues[13] also documented increased dermal angiogenesis with the diode laser treatment. Frew and colleagues[14] evaluated the use of the diode laser component in a split comparison study in which half of the area was treated with all 3 components of the TriActive system and the other half was treated without the diode laser. An 83% improvement in cellulite was reported in the laser-added side in comparison with an average 17% improvement on the non-laser-treated side. Therefore they concluded that the diode laser component significantly contributed to clinical improvement.

Kulick and colleagues[15] investigated the efficacy of the SmoothShapes (Eleme Medical, Merrimack, NH, USA) device for the treatment of cellulite by using a 3D imaging system (Vectra; Canfield Scientific). SmoothShapes is a dual wavelength, 915-nm and 650-nm, laser device that is combined with a vacuum-assisted mechanical massage. The basis of these wavelength selections is based on adipose samples treated with a 635-nm light from a 10-mW diode laser, which showed emptying of fat from these cells.[16] Then the 915-nm wavelength penetrates into the tissue and is preferentially absorbed by lipids, causing a thermal effect. The temperature inside the adipocyte is elevated by up to 6°C. The 650-nm wavelength is thought to modify the permeability of the fat cell membranes, allowing expressed fat to move into the interstitial space, without ever destroying the adipocyte cell membrane. The fat is moved into the interstitial space and lymphatic system for elimination with the aid of mechanical rollers and mild suction. Without the use of rollers and suction, the fat would return into the adipocyte within 45 minutes. This device also has multiple handpieces for different body surfaces.

A study of 20 women who were treated in the posterior-lateral thigh area 2 times per week for 4 weeks was conducted. Treatment time was 15 minutes per thigh and the maximum energy settings were used. Suction settings were medium intensity initially and then increased to maximum as tolerated. During the treatment, all target areas had an increase in average skin temperature after treatment of about 5.9°C. Ninety-four percent of the patients thought their cellulite was improved and remained improved 6 months after the last treatment. The 3D imaging analysis showed an 82% improvement at 1 month, 76% improvement at 3 months, and 76% improvement at 6 months. Six months after treatment, the average surface elevation was 2.3 mm (range, 0.63–5.6 mm) and the average flattening was 4.9 mm (range, 1.4–7.8 mm). The average volume change was 84-mL reduction (range, 17.4–152 mL).

SURGICAL TREATMENT OPTIONS

Surgical treatment options for cellulite consist of mechanical destruction of dermal septae via either subcision or laser-assisted devices.[17]

Subcision uses a 16- or 18-gauge needle or a blade inserted into the subcutaneous adipose layer, parallel to the epidermis, to break the septae separating the fat lobules. By cutting the septae, it is hypothesized that the structure of the subcutaneous fat producing the cellulite is altered, thus leading to less tethering of the underlying connective tissue to the epidermis. Hexsel and Mazzuco[18] studied 232 cellulite patients treated with subcision in the thigh and buttock areas. Of patients, 78.8% reported being satisfied with the results achieved after one session. Twenty-three patients who were seen in a 2 or greater year follow-up visit had lasting results,[18] which purports the mechanism of action of cutting cellulite septae for improvement.

Laser-induced lipolysis can cause a reduction in adipose deposits by physically disrupting cellular membranes as well as causing a thermal coagulation of dermal collagen, resulting in clinical skin tightening. O'Dey and colleagues reported the use of a 940-nm diode laser for adipose tissue ablation. They purported that the 940-nm wavelength selectively targeted both adipose tissue and water with a penetration depth of several millimeters. The water in the connective tissue septae was suspected to be responsible for some collateral damage leading to the vaporization of adipose cells.

The neodymium-doped yttrium aluminum garnet (Nd:YAG) laser has been used extensively for adipose tissue removal and now for cellulite treatment. The Nd:YAG laser uses a short yet high-peak power to destroy adipose cells via a photo-acoustic effect. At the same time the thermal energy also coagulates tissue to achieve hemostasis and subsequent collagen tightening. Kim and Geronemus[19] showed that there is an energy-dependent relationship between volume reduction during laser lipolysis with a 1064-nm Nd:YAG. They also demonstrated that subdermal bands were ruptured by the thermal effect, which clinically manifested as a release of retracted skin areas.

McBean and Katz studied the application of a sequentially firing 1064- and 1320-nm Nd:YAG laser device for lipolysis and skin tightening. India ink–tattooed areas were used to assess topographic skin tightening. They reported a 76% to 100% improvement in adiposities in 85% of subjects and 51% to 75% improvement in 15% of subjects. In 5 patients with India ink tattoo maps, an 18% decrease in surface area was seen, implying a skin tightening effect. Histologic samples taken showed new collagen formation compared with baseline.[20]

Cellulaze (Cynosure) is a laser device that uses a 1440-nm Nd:YAG fiber with a novel delivery

Table 1
Absorption of 1440-nm wavelength compared with other wavelengths

Wavelengths	Fatty Tissue	Water
1064 nm	1	1
924 nm	2.8	1.4
980 nm	1.7	3.6
1320 nm	5.9	11.5
1440 nm	127	252

system to target the structural components of cellulite. The technology incorporates a unique SideLight Side-Firing Fiber as well as a ThermaGuide thermal sensing system for safer treatments. The 1440-nm wavelength is highly absorbed in adipose tissue, which is composed of 75% fat, 20% water, and 5% proteins. The 1440-nm wavelength is absorbed by adipose tissue 127 times greater and absorbed by water 252 times greater than the 1064-nm wavelength (**Table 1**).

The side-firing mechanism fires laser energy bidirectionally, forward from the laser fiber tip as well as orthogonal to this direction, simultaneously. Up to 40% of the energy is delivered through the distal end of fiber and about 60% is delivered through the side of fiber (**Fig. 3**). The ThermaGuide technology provides the ability to deliver acute thermal damage in a safe manner. The set temperature threshold is at 45 to 47°C and, once that temperature is reached, the ThermaGuide will give an audible signal and stop the laser from firing. For this procedure, a mapping template is used to outline 5 × 5 cm² squares. "Hills" are marked in green and "valleys" marked in red that are at least 3 × 3 cm² (**Fig. 4**). Tumescent anesthesia is used. Sixty to 80 mL of Klein tumescent anesthesia per 5 × 5 cm² is recommended. Using the laser settings of 10 W of power, 25 Hz repetition rate, and 1000 μs maximum pulse width, 1000 J is to be delivered per 5 × 5 cm². These amounts include the energy needed to

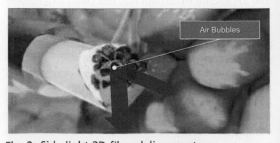

Fig. 3. Side light 3D fiber delivery system.

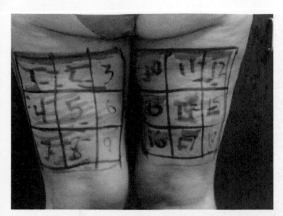

Fig. 4. Cellulaze preoperative markings.

deplane fat, subcise septa, and heat the dermis. The subcutaneous temperature should be kept at less than 47°C and the surface temperature, measured by infrared thermometer, should be kept at 38 to 40°C.

The first step involves deplaning of fat cells to minimize expansion of tissue that causes bulging. This disruption of the adipose tissue allows contouring of raised areas of bulging fat or, "hills" and is performed in the fat layer. The cannula is inserted at an approximate depth of 1 to 2 cm with the fiber pointing down and reciprocated back and forth in a fanlike motion until the recommended Joules are reached. Next, thermal subcision of septae is commenced to target the depressed "valleys" clinically. This thermal subcision is done with the fiber pointed sideways about 3 to 5 mm below the skin surface. Finally, there is heating of the superficial layer to promote skin thickening and tightening for a smooth even dermis.

DiBernardo[21] reported that the use of a 1440-nm laser subdermally could disrupt and reduce herniated fat in the dermis, through a process of tissue coagulation. They demonstrated ultrasound evidence of a 25% increase in skin thickness and a 29% decrease in skin laxity, which was maintained at 1 year.

Katz and colleagues[22] conducted a study of 15 patients treated with this technology to assess the safety and efficacy of a single treatment with the Nd:YAG 1440-nm wavelength laser. 2D and 3D photography (Vectra) were used to evaluate clinical outcomes, such as a change in dimples and contour irregularities. Patients had grades II to III cellulite. Adverse events were evaluated at 1 week, and then at 2, 3, and 6 months posttreatment. Photos using 2D photography and 3D images were taken at baseline, 2, 3, and 6 months posttreatment. The average decrease of dimple (valley) depth (based on absolute dimple depth value) was 42% at 3 months (n = 24, P = .00015) and 49% at 6 months (n = 24, P = .00032). Of patients, 62% showed improvement at 3 months and 66% of patients showed improvement at 6 months (**Figs. 5–7**).

TREATMENT RESISTANCE/COMPLICATIONS

Depending on the grade and severity, some cellulite patients may see a lesser degree of improvement. It is important in the consultation to frame patient expectations. Noninvasive treatments require multiple treatments as well as possible interval maintenance treatments. Resistant cases could be due to severity of the case or undertreatment of the area. When using laser, radiofrequency, or ultrasound devices, it is important not to deliver excessive fluences as this could lead to unwarranted treatment complications and or thermal damage.

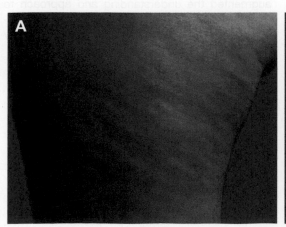
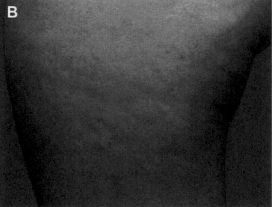

Fig. 5. Clinical photos—baseline and 6-month follow-up: (*A*) baseline; (*B*) 6 months after.

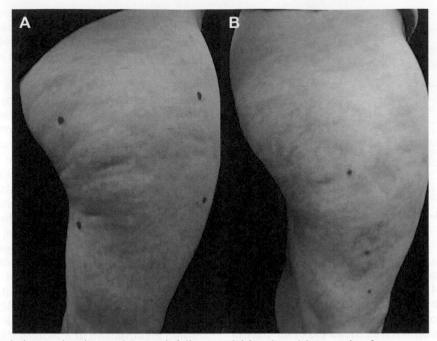

Fig. 6. Clinical photos—baseline and 6-month follow-up: (*A*) baseline; (*B*) 6 months after.

EVALUATION OF OUTCOME AND LONG-TERM RECOMMENDATIONS

It is important to see all patients in follow-up. Measurements to be taken include dimple severity, circumference, and overall laxity. Patient satisfaction should also be assessed. For surgical patients follow-up at 3 and 6 months can provide enough

Baseline

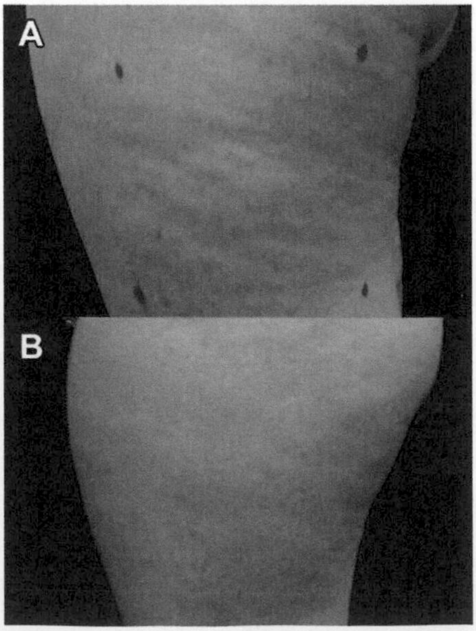

6 month post op

Fig. 7. Clinical photos—baseline and 6-month follow-up: (*A*) baseline; (*B*) 6 months after.

healing time and remodeling to assess improvement. The use of traditional 2D imaging as well as 3D imaging can augment follow-up visits and patient satisfaction as well as give an objective comparison from baseline.

SUMMARY

Cellulite is a well-documented condition and, although many treatment options have been purported, few have lasting clinical results. This historically notorious problem now has a modern resurgence of treatment technology. The use of laser- and light-based devices, in both a noninvasive and a minimally invasive fashion, has augmented the understanding and approach to the treatment of cellulite. Understanding the structural components that underpin cellulite anatomy allows for a more specific targeting approach.

REFERENCES

1. Avram MM. Cellulite: a review of its physiology and treatment. J Cosmet Laser Ther 2004;6(4):181–5.
2. Rossi AB, Vergnanini AL. Cellulite: a review. J Eur Acad Dermatol Venereol 2000;14(4):251–62.
3. Nurnberger F, Muller G. So-called cellulite: an invented disease. J Dermatol Surg Oncol 1978;4(3):221–9.
4. Collis N, Elliot LA, Sharpe C, et al. Cellulite treatment: a myth or reality: a prospective randomized, controlled trial of two therapies, endermologie and

aminophylline cream. Plast Reconstr Surg 1999; 104(4):1110–4 [discussion: 1115–7].

5. Am Kligman A, Pagnoni A, Stroudemayer T. Topical retinol improves cellulite. J Dermatolog Treat 1999; 10(2):119–25.

6. Anderson RR, Farinelli W, Laubach H, et al. Selective photothermolysis of lipid-rich tissues: a free electron laser study. Lasers Surg Med 2006;38(10):913–9.

7. Nootheti PK, Magpantay A, Yosowitz G, et al. A single center, randomized, comparative, prospective clinical study to determine the efficacy of the VelaSmooth system versus the Triactive system for the treatment of cellulite. Lasers Surg Med 2006;38(10):908–12.

8. Draelos ZD, Marenus KD. Cellulite. Etiology and purported treatment. Dermatol Surg 1997;23(12): 1177–81.

9. Alster TS, Tanzi EL. Cellulite treatment using a novel combination radiofrequency, infrared light, and mechanical tissue manipulation device. J Cosmet Laser Ther 2005;7(2):81–5.

10. Sadick N, Magro C. A study evaluating the safety and efficacy of the VelaSmooth system in the treatment of cellulite. J Cosmet Laser Ther 2007;9(1):15–20.

11. Emilia del Pino M, Rosado RH, Azuela A, et al. Effect of controlled volumetric tissue heating with radiofrequency on cellulite and the subcutaneous tissue of the buttocks and thighs. J Drugs Dermatol 2006; 5(8):714–22.

12. Goldberg DJ, Fazeli A, Berlin AL. Clinical, laboratory, and MRI analysis of cellulite treatment with a unipolar radiofrequency device. Dermatol Surg 2008;34(2):204–9 [discussion: 209].

13. Schindl A, Merwald H, Schindl L, et al. Direct stimulatory effect of low-intensity 670 nm laser irradiation on human endothelial cell proliferation. Br J Dermatol 2003;148(2):334–6.

14. Frew K, Katz B, The efficacy of a diode laser with contact cooling and suction (TriActive System) in the treatment of cellilite. Presented at the 13th Congress of the European Academy of Dermatology and Venereology. Florence.

15. Kulick MI. Evaluation of a noninvasive, dual-wavelength laser-suction and massage device for the regional treatment of cellulite. Plast Reconstr Surg 2010;125(6):1788–96.

16. Neira R, Toledo L, Arroyave J, et al. Low-level laser-assisted liposuction: the Neira 4 L technique. Clin Plast Surg 2006;33(1):117–27, vii.

17. van Vliet M, Ortiz A, Avram MM, et al. An assessment of traditional and novel therapies for cellulite. J Cosmet Laser Ther 2005;7(1):7–10.

18. Hexsel DM, Mazzuco R. Subcision: a treatment for cellulite. Int J Dermatol 2000;39(7):539–44.

19. Kim KH, Geronemus RG. Laser lipolysis using a novel 1,064 nm Nd:YAG Laser. Dermatol Surg 2006;32(2):241–8 [discussion: 247].

20. McBean JC, Katz BE. A pilot study of the efficacy of a 1,064 and 1,320 nm sequentially firing Nd:YAG laser device for lipolysis and skin tightening. Lasers Surg Med 2009;41(10):779–84.

21. DiBernardo BE. Treatment of cellulite using a 1440-nm pulsed laser with one-year follow-up. Aesthet Surg J 2011;31(3):328–41.

22. Katz BE, Quantitative & Qualitative Evaluation of the Efficacy of a1440 nm Nd:YAG laser with novel bi-directional optical fiber in the treatment of cellulite as measured by 3-dimensional surface imaging. J Drugs Dermatol, in press.

Future Directions in Cutaneous Laser Surgery

Sabrina Guillen Fabi, MD[a],*, Andrei I. Metelitsa, MD, FRCPC[b]

KEYWORDS

- Laser • Cutaneous lasers • Wavelength • Picosecond • 1565 nm • 1940 nm • 1210 nm

KEY POINTS

- Numerous innovations have been made in cutaneous laser surgery.
- In addition to perfecting already established treatment modalities, the scope of the field is continuously expanding, with new clinical indications being added to the armamentarium of laser experts.
- More selective treatment of existing targets ensures improved efficacy, with fewer side effects and treatment sessions.
- The identification of new targets allows for more effective treatment of common cutaneous conditions.
- Adjunctive applications optimize treatment results and the diagnostic acumen of clinicians.
- Future applications will include waveforms beyond those in the visible light and infrared spectrum, such as microwaves, ultrasound waves, and radiofrequency.

INTRODUCTION

Laser therapy has advanced in the treatment of various skin lesions and conditions, benefiting both patients and physicians. In the past 45 years there have also been important advances in the understanding of cutaneous physiology and laser technology, leading to a plethora of laser devices on the market enabling specialized treatment of multiple skin disorders. Developments of new, more precise lasers and targeted therapy aim to provide safer outcomes, with optimal lesion clearance and improved patient satisfaction.

Laser therapy has revolutionized the treatment of both classic and aesthetic dermatology. Many conditions are routinely, sometimes exclusively, treated with lasers, such as vascular and pigmented lesions, acne scars, tattoos, rhytides, and acne and precancerous lesions when combined

with a photosensitizer. However, many cutaneous lesions and conditions do not always completely resolve, causing disappointment to both doctors and patients.

This article presents an overview of the future course of cutaneous laser therapy and technology. To enhance efficacy and specificity of treatment, new wavelengths directed at both old and new targets are on the horizon. New applications, including the use of lasers to aid in the detection of skin cancers and to enhance drug delivery, are being used and investigated. A trend toward combining different lasers and light sources to optimize results continues, with different laser combinations being used as new technologies emerge. To reach a broader population, advancements in at-home devices have been made for which, although not a replacement for existing laser devices that create a deeper and more

Financial Disclosures: Dr Fabi is a consultant/speaker for Ulthera, Inc and Lumenis. Dr Metelitsa is a consultant for Cutera, Cynosure and Clarion.

a Goldman, Butterwick, Fitzpatrick, Groff, & Fabi, Cosmetic Laser Dermatology, 9339 Genesee Avenue, Suite 300, San Diego, CA 92121, USA; b Institute for Skin Advancement, University of Calgary, Suite 203, 4935 40 Avenue NW, Calgary, Alberta, Canada
* Corresponding author.
E-mail address: sfabi@gbkderm.com

Dermatol Clin 32 (2014) 61–69
http://dx.doi.org/10.1016/j.det.2013.09.004

significant level of injury, there is a demand. There is also no denying that the future includes waveforms beyond those in the visible light and infrared spectrum, such as microwaves, ultrasound waves, and radiofrequency.

NEW WAVELENGTHS, NEW TARGETS

Anderson and colleagues proposed the theory of selective photothermolysis (SP) in 1983. The concept refers to the precise targeting of a structure or tissue using a specific wavelength of light with the intention of absorbing light into that target area alone, the goal being that sufficient energy is absorbed by the target, leaving the surrounding tissue relatively unaffected.[1,2]

For years commonly targeted chromophores have included hemoglobin, deoxyhemoglobin, melanin, and water, which have allowed the successful treatment of vascular and pigmented lesions and conditions, as well as laser hair removal, the improvement of acne scar remodeling, and rhytid improvement. However, of the many available laser wavelengths in the marketplace, none have ever specifically targeted the sebaceous glands involved in sebaceous hyperplasia and the pathophysiology of acne.

Until now dermatologists have relied on topical photodynamic therapy (PDT), which requires the interaction of an exogenous photosensitizer, an activating light source, and the presence of oxygen, to target sebaceous glands. A topical non-photosensitizing prodrug, 5-aminolevulinic acid (ALA), and methylaminolevulinic acid, its more lipophilic methylated counterpart, are preferentially absorbed by and metabolized within sebaceous glands, as well as superficial melanin, superficial cutaneous vasculature, and rapidly proliferating cells, producing highly photoactive protoporphyrin IX (PpIX).[3,4] PpIX excitation occurs with a light source of an appropriate wavelength, leading to the formation of cytotoxic singlet oxygen and other reactive oxygen species, with subsequent target cell death and localized oxidative stress.[5] Secondary vascular damage also results from vasoconstriction, thrombosis, ischemia, and subsequent necrosis of the vessels associated with the target.

Although not specific in treating sebaceous glands alone, well-controlled clinical studies have demonstrated the ability of pulsed lasers, specifically pulsed dye laser and intense pulsed light (IPL), to successfully target cutaneous sebaceous glands via photodynamic and photothermal mechanisms, leading to the improvement of sebaceous hyperplasia.[6,7] Several randomized controlled clinical trials have also demonstrated statistically significant reductions in inflammatory lesions of acne vulgaris using PDT,[8–12] improvement which is thought to partly contribute to the apoptosis of sebocytes from PDT.[13]

Wavelength 1720 nm and Sebaceous Glands

An SP in vitro study to determine wavelengths potentially able to target sebaceous glands was performed by Sakamoto and colleagues.[14] Absorption peaks near 1210, 1728, 1760, 2306, and 2346 nm were found with the use of a free-electron laser pulsed at an infrared $CH(2)$ vibrational absorption wavelength band on natural and artificially prepared sebum. Laser-induced heating at 1710 and 1720 nm was about 1.5-fold higher in human sebaceous glands than in water. Histology of skin samples exposed to pulses of approximately 1700 nm and 100 to 125 milliseconds showed evidence of selective thermal damage to sebaceous glands. With the use of wavelengths that more specifically target sebum, the investigators hypothesized that SP of sebaceous glands, another part of hair follicles, may equate to the success of permanent hair removal via laser.[14]

In a pilot clinical study to evaluate the efficacy of a novel 1720-nm laser in the treatment of sebaceous hyperplasia, 4 patients underwent a test spot, followed by 2 full treatment sessions using the 1720-nm laser (Del Mar Medical Technologies, Del Mar, CA, USA). A 400-μm fiber, with a mean fluence of 45 J/cm^2, spot size of 750 μm, and pulse duration of 50 milliseconds was used to deliver the energy. The desired end point was a change from pretreatment granular yellow appearance to a creamy-white smooth surface. Damage to adjacent normal skin showed no change until the pulse duration exceeded twice that of the sebaceous hyperplasia. A panel of 3 independent dermatologists blinded to the date of the photographs evaluated the photos and scored them based on a global assessment comprising: (1) lesion diameter, (2) lesion height, and (3) lesion color. Many of the lesions resolved almost completely after a single treatment, and no additional treatment was required. There was a mean global improvement of 3.9 (3 = 51%–75% improvement and 4 = 76%–99% improvement). Crusts were noted by all patients, which resolved within 10 days.[15]

Complete heating of the sebaceous gland and sparing of the surrounding skin offered by the investigated device resulted in clinically apparent improvement with a minimum of adverse effects. Further studies are warranted, with larger sample sizes, to investigate the efficacy of this novel wavelength and possible future wavelengths in the SP of sebaceous glands and its impact in the improvement of sebaceous hyperplasia, ectopic sebaceous glands, acne vulgaris, and laser hair removal.

Perhaps there is also hope beyond the use of lasers for SP of sebaceous glands, such as that seen with microfocused ultrasound with visualization (MFU-V) for the treatment of moderate to severe facial acne. Although the mechanism of action remains unclear, it is hypothesized that with the use of 1.5-mm and 1-mm depth probes, focal thermal coagulation points are being delivered into sebaceous glands, rendering them not as active. In a pilot study in which 10 subjects received 3 treatments, 14 days apart with MFU-V, a significant decrease in sebum, as measured by a sebumeter (Courage-Khazaka, Cologne, Germany), was noted over the forehead, cheeks, and chin 60 days after treatment. Eighty percent of subjects had a decrease in total acne lesion count at 60 days, and 100% of subjects showed a decrease at 180 days after the last treatment. Data from this pilot trial suggest that MFU-V may prove to be a promising novel treatment option to improve acne clearance in those with moderate to severe inflammatory acne.[16]

NEW WAVELENGTHS, OLD TARGETS

With advances in the understanding, theory, and technology of lasers and related energy devices over the past 5 decades, the field has also been witness to the evolution of multiple lasers, with various wavelengths. For instance, in the past continuous-wave lasers such as the argon, tunable dye, krypton, and copper vapor lasers were used to target hemoglobin, but because these lasers do not restrict damage to the targeted chromophore, there was a high prevalence of dyschromia and scarring. New devices were developed that had high chromophore specificity and minimized these risks, including pulsed dye lasers (577, 585, and 595 nm), long-pulsed alexandrite lasers (755 nm), pulsed diode lasers (in the range of 800–900 nm), long-pulsed 1064-nm Nd:YAG lasers, and IPL sources.[1,2]

Although many wavelengths are available in the marketplace, new wavelengths continue to emerge to more selectively target established chromophores such as fat, vasculature, pigment, and collagen, with the goal of increasing the efficacy and safety of treatment.

Wavelength 1210 nm

Absorption peaks near 915, 1210, 1400, 1720, and 2346 nm have been demonstrated for lipids.[17] A study to evaluate the histologic changes over time of a novel noninvasive treatment with a 1210-nm laser with surface cooling, to more

selectively target fat, was performed on 8 patients before abdominoplasty.[18] Skin evaluations and blood monitoring were tracked for safety. Postabdominoplasty tissue was evaluated histologically at 2 days, 1 week, and 1, 3, and 6 months after laser treatment with energy doses ranging from 120 to 200 J/cm^2 and from 220 to 480 J/cm^2 for 40-second and 160-second pulses, respectively. A decrease in nitroblue tetrazolium chloride staining showed damaged zones, predominantly in the hypodermis, approaching 6 mm in thickness. Laser damage to the lipid barrier membrane was confirmed by a decrease in perilipin staining, and caspase staining confirmed apoptotic adipocytes at the periphery of necrotic tissue. Chronic inflammatory cells were still present at 6 months after laser treatment. Damage to the lower dermis was higher for the 40-second pulse than for the 160-second pulse. The investigators concluded that significant zones of fat reduction in hypodermal necrosis could be achieved, while including or avoiding damage to the lower dermis depending on the settings used. Clearance of the damaged adipocytes proved slow, with residual damage still present at 6 months.[18]

A clinical trial was performed to evaluate the use of the 1210-nm wavelength (ORlight, Potters Bar, UK) for fat preservation,[19] as the investigators describe this wavelength as being capable of selective photothermostimulation (PSP), a concept whereby the wavelength has the ability to stimulate adipocytes and mesenchymal cells of the subcutaneous tissue. One hundred two patients were treated with the 1210-nm diode laser and followed. Samples of aspirated tissue were sent for histologic analysis to determine whether any alteration of adipocytes occurred with treatment. Histologic analyses revealed a 98% preservation of aspirated adipocytes. The investigators hypothesize that this selective PSP and preservation of the integrity of adipocytes makes this laser wavelength ideal when performing laser-assisted liposculpture followed by fat grafting or breast reconstruction.[19]

There may be a place for the addition of another wavelength that has a greater absorption affinity for lipid-rich tissue than the wavelengths of lasers presently on the market. Further studies, with larger sample sizes, will help determine the benefit of this novel wavelength in laser-assisted lipoplasty and, perhaps, the removal of large lipomas.

1565-nm Erbium-Doped Laser

The development of fractional photothermolysis (FP) is a milestone in the history of laser technology and cutaneous resurfacing. FP refers to the creation of pixilated columnar zones of thermal injury, referred to as microthermal treatment zones, which are delivered to the dermis, with resultant coagulation necrosis followed by collagen remodeling and synthesis. Selective injury of the dermis with relative or absolute sparing of the epidermis was established and termed "nonablative." Unlike traditional nonablative infrared lasers, nonablative fractionated lasers (NAFL) treat only a fraction of the skin, being able to leave up to a maximum of 95% of the skin uninvolved.[20] This targeting allows the undamaged surrounding tissue to act as a reservoir of viable tissue, permitting rapid epidermal repair. In 2003, the first NAFL was introduced to the market based on the concept of FP, namely the fractionated 1550-nm erbium-doped "fraxel" laser, now called the Fraxel Re:Store (Fraxel Re:Store, Solta Medical, Hayward, CA, USA).

NAFL can be used to treat a variety of conditions, including fine lines and wrinkles, dyschromia, striae, and scars. The benefits are minimal downtime and relatively low risk of adverse effects. Since the inception of NAFL, a variety of NAFLs with wavelengths in the near-infrared range have surfaced as a result its popularity, including the Q-Switched 1064-nm Nd:YAG (HarmonyXL Alma Lasers, Buffalo Grove, IL, USA), the 1440-nm Nd:YAG (Affirm; Cynosure Inc, Westford, MA, USA and Palomar Starlux, Artisan, Icon; Palomar Medical Technologies, Burlington, MA, USA), 1440/1320-nm Nd:YAG (Affirm Multiplex; Cynosure), 1440-nm diode (Clear and Brilliant System; Solta Medical), 1540-nm erbium:glass (Palomar Starlux, Artisan, Icon; Palomar Medical Technologies), 1927-nm thulium (Fraxel Re:Store Dual; Solta Medical), and 1927-nm diode (Clear and Brilliant Perméa handpiece on the Clear and Brilliant System; Solta Medical).

A new NAFL with no disposable tips, with a handpiece that allows real-time "cool-scanning" in a stamping fashion, was recently approved by the Food and Drug Administration (FDA) (M22 [ResurFx module]; Lumenis, Inc, San Jose, CA, USA). Infrared laser energy at 1565 nm has a slightly lower absorption coefficient for water than that of 1550 nm (9/cm and 8/cm, respectively), leading to marginally greater dermal penetration.[21] A wide variety of shapes, densities, and sizes of patterns are offered, ranging from 5 to 18 mm. Energy level ranges from 10 to 70 mJ with density ranging from 50 to 500 spots/cm^2. Preliminary results of a 2-center trial treating a total of 30 subjects with visible rhytides (Fitzpatrick Wrinkle Score of 3–6) and/or striae alba (present for >1 year), who received a single-pass treatment monthly for 3 consecutive treatments, shows appreciable results and high patient satisfaction. Future studies to determine its efficacy in the treatment of scars and dyschromia, as well as to compare its performance with that of other NAFL devices, will optimize its application.

1940-nm Nonablative Fractionated Laser

1940 nm is a novel wavelength that has a higher absorption coefficient for water than other nonablative wavelengths (1410–1550 nm), and is weaker than ablative wavelengths. A new fractional 1940-nm laser comprises thulium rod pumped by a pulsed alexandrite laser. The fractional patterns are generated by 3 separate hand pieces (2 dot and 1 grid geometries) whereby a larger beam is broken up into smaller microbeams by a diffractive microlens system. Its depth of penetration extends approximately 200 μm deep to the surface. In a pilot trial of 11 patients with facial photodamage,[22] patients received 3 full-face treatments, carried out in 2 passes, 4 to 6 weeks apart, using topical anesthesia and cold-air cooling for patient comfort. Outcome assessments included changes in pigment, rhytides, laxity, texture, and elastosis. Three months after the last treatment, mean texture scores were unchanged, rhytides were reduced by 15% ($P = .05$), and pigment improved by 30% ($P = .05$). Downtime from the procedure ranged from 3 to 5 days and the only adverse event reported was mild vesiculation in 2 patients.[22]

ENHANCED DRUG DELIVERY

It is known that the epidermal permeability barrier, primarily constituted by the stratum corneum, limits the uptake of topically applied drugs. Pixilated microchannels that are created by ablative fractionated lasers (AFxL) can increase skin permeability, and have been shown to facilitate transdermal delivery of drugs both in vitro and in vivo.[23–26] Waibel and Wulkan[27] most recently reported the synergistic benefit of laser-assisted delivery of triamcinolone and 5-fluorouracil for the improvement of hypertrophic and keloidal scars using AFxL. Various studies are also being conducted on the pretreatment of skin with an AFxL to enhance the delivery of topical photosensitizers to optimize treatment of both precancerous and cancerous cutaneous lesions. In addition to drugs, transdermal delivery of adipose-derived stem cells has more recently been shown to be successful when skin was pretreated with an AFxL (erbium:YAG [Er:YAG] laser, Profile; Sciton, Inc, Palo Alto, CA, USA) using a 1000-μm depth at 22% density.[28–30] Potential future applications of this approach might include wound healing, as well as aesthetic indications.

NEW TARGETS, OLD WAVELENGTHS
Eccrine and Apocrine Glands

Primary axillary hyperhidrosis and osmidrosis typically begin at puberty, and are distressing conditions characterized by an odoriferous smell, profuse sweating, and, occasionally, staining of clothes. Treatment options are limited by duration of effect, side effects, and/or by effectiveness. There are few isolated retrospective and case studies reporting the use of Nd:YAG lasers subdermally in the treatment of hyperhidrosis.[27,28] Most recently Yanes[31] presented results on the use of the 924/927 nm diode laser subdermally, via a 1.5-mm diameter flexible fiber, to selectively destroy axillary sweat glands before aspiration and curettage. When a long-pulsed 800-nm diode laser was used externally for 5 cycles in a randomized controlled half-side comparison study, no significant decrease in sweat rate was observed.[32]

Less invasive energy-based, nonlaser treatment options for the treatment of axillary hyperhidrosis have become much more common in recent years. Although microwaves are not commonly used in cutaneous surgery, they are able to focus heat at the interface between the skin and subcutaneous tissue, causing irreversible thermal necrosis of both apocrine and eccrine glands.[33] In 2011 a microwave device was approved by the FDA for the treatment of primary axillary hyperhidrosis.[34] In a multicenter, randomized, sham-controlled, blinded trial, a total of 81 patients underwent 2 treatments, 2 weeks apart, and were allowed to undergo a third treatment within 30 days if they still had excess sweating after 2 sessions. Thirty days after treatment, the active group had a response rate of 89% (72 of 81) and the sham group had a responder rate of 54% (21 of 39) ($P<.001$). Treatment efficacy was stable from 3 months (74%) to 12 months (69%), when follow-up ended. The most common adverse events were soreness and swelling at the treated site, which typically resolved within 9 days. Additional side effects included altered limb sensation, pain, blisters, rash, axillary nodules, and compensatory swelling, all of which resolved except the altered limb sensation in 1 patient.[34]

In addition to microwaves, more recently MFU-V has been investigated for the treatment of axillary hyperhidrosis. In a randomized, double-blind controlled trial, 12 of 20 hyperhidrotic adults with Hyperhidrosis Disease Severity Scale scores of 3 or 4 underwent 2 treatments, 30 days apart.[35] The sham group (8 of 20) received treatment with the energy turned to 0 J. Patients were followed for 4 months, and a response rate of 67% to 83% ($P<.005$) was seen across all post-treatment time points for the active group, versus 0% for the sham group. Given the positive results of this pilot study, additional histologic studies are being undertaken as well as a pivotal clinical trial.

Optical Nanomaterials

Optical nanomaterials present a promising platform for targeted molecular imaging of cancer biomarkers and its photodestruction. Owing to the development of novel nanomaterials, such as gold, silver, and carbon, as light absorption agents, photothermal therapy is presently being used for cancer therapy in different medical specialties as a minimally invasive treatment modality to target malignant cells.[36,37] As these nanoparticles are easily internalized by cells, as demonstrated by imaging using both reflected bright-light optical microscopy and surface-enhanced Raman spectroscopy (SERS), the particles have proved to be detectable inside cells under a wide window of excitation wavelengths, ranging from visible to near infrared (NIR). Their high sensitivity and NIR availability make this class of SERS nanotags a promising candidate for noninvasive imaging and targeting of cancer cells.

In a study comparing the effect of ALA and ALA combined with gold nanoparticles (ALA-AuNPs) for PDT on human cervical cancer cell lines, ALA-AuNP resulted in greater cytotoxicity and cell injury in comparison with ALA alone.[38]

These nanomaterials are currently being investigated in laser cutaneous surgery to more effectively target cutaneous structures and increase the efficacy of treatment, and may possibly play a role in the treatment of cutaneous malignancies as well as targeting sebaceous glands for the treatment of acne.

NEW APPLICATIONS
Diagnosis of Skin Cancer

With continually rising incidence rates of skin cancer in North America, the importance of early detection is absolutely critical. A novel Raman spectroscopy system utilizes a near-infrared 785-nm laser beam and scans the biochemical constituents of the skin based on molecular vibration. Within seconds, this system scans for 21 biomarkers and provides very specific spectral patterns identifying biochemical composition of the tissue, and allows clinicians to determine whether a lesion is truly malignant. In fact, over the past 6 years nearly 1000 skin lesions have been examined, with the most recent study showing a sensitivity of 99% in differentiating malignant and premalignant skin lesions from benign ones.[39] A commercial product, Verisante Aura (Verisante Technology, Inc, Vancouver, BC, Canada) is already approved by Health Canada and is claimed to reduce the number of unnecessary biopsies by 50% to 100%.

NEW PROPERTIES
Picosecond

Tattoo removal has graduated from the days of nonselective ablation with the carbon dioxide and argon-ion continuous-wave lasers to the present SP with quality-switched (QS) lasers. Adverse effects such as scarring and dyspigmentation have been greatly reduced because water is no longer the target chromophore.

Furthermore, the generally smaller tattoo pigments possess thermal relaxation times of less than 10 nanoseconds, requiring treatment with lasers possessing even shorter pulse durations. At present, currently available QS lasers reliably release high-powered pulses in the range of nanoseconds. This fast heating causes rapid expansion, fragmentation, and resultant formation of acoustic waves, along with photothermal effects, which ultimately destroy the tattoo particles. However, while the advances in laser science are certainly impressive, the art of tattoo removal is still far from perfect, especially because removal of professional tattoos often necessitates 8 or more treatment sessions.

The use of laser pulses of sub-nanosecond duration, called picosecond pulses, is able to more effectively confine the energy to the tattoo particle, resulting in a more effective photoacoustic breakup of the target. Analyses of heat and stress evolution in a tattoo target have been performed by solving the heat-transfer equation and the acoustic-propagation equation, using laser pulses of 50 picoseconds to 50 nanoseconds, which indicate that picosecond pulses result in a greater thermal response of the tattoo target. In addition, these pulses create mechanical stress that is not possible with nanosecond pulses.[40] Picosecond lasers also require the use of lower treatment fluences, thus decreasing the risk of adverse reactions.

Technical challenges in bringing the technology to fruition have kept the picosecond lasers out of the aesthetic laser market. Recently, lasers that can be operated in practitioner's offices have begun to be investigated. Several prospective trials have assessed the efficacy of a novel picosecond 755-nm alexandrite laser (Cynosure, Inc, Westford, MA, USA). In a study of 15 patients, all

12 of the patients who completed the study noted greater than 75% clearance after an average of 4.25 treatment sessions.[41] Pulse duration was reported to be in the range of 500 to 900 picoseconds, with fluence ranging between 2.1 and 4.1 J/cm^2, and spot sizes from 2.5 to 3.5 mm. Overall, treatments were reported to be safe and very effective, and tattoos cleared 50% more rapidly than historical controls. Another study of 12 tattoos containing blue and/or green pigment reported the use of a picosecond laser with variable pulse widths of 750 to 900 picoseconds, spot sizes ranging from 3.0 to 3.6 mm, and fluence ranging from 2.0 to 2.83 J/cm^2.[42] Following only 1 treatment, 11 of the 12 treated tattoos had achieved greater than 75% clearance of the blue and/or green pigment, with more than two-thirds of treated tattoos approaching closer to 100% clearance.

In addition to trials on the treatment of tattoos, studies investigating the picosecond 755-nm alexandrite laser (Cynosure) on facial scarring and striae using a defractive lens show promising results.[43,44] Additional studies are under way for its use in melasma. In the future, additional wavelengths delivering picosecond pulse durations will aid in more effectively treating red-colored tattoos.

HOME DEVICES

Over the past several years, several home-based cosmetic devices have been introduced to the market. These miniaturized devices are designed to address a variety of indications, including photorejuvenation, acne, hair growth, and hair removal.[45] Although underpowered when compared with their in-office counterparts, these devices appeal to patients given their ability to perform treatments in the privacy of one's home at a significantly lower cost. These lasers also incorporate specific safety features to ensure that "nonprofessional" operators can use them with ease.

One of the first fractional, photorejuvenation devices to be launched was the PaloVia Skin Renewing Laser (Palomar Medical Technologies, Burlington, MA, USA). This hand-held, nonablative diode laser (1410 nm, 15 mJ, 10-millisecond pulse duration) has been cleared by the FDA for reduction of fine lines and wrinkles around the eyes, with 2 of the studies showing improvement of at least 1 grade in facial wrinkle score in up to 90% of the patients after 1 month of daily treatment. Another home-based, fractional diode device (1435 nm, 1.2 W) is the Philips Reaura (Philips, Amsterdam, the Netherlands), with initial studies claiming rejuvenation effects in 8 weeks following twice-weekly application. In addition, new in-home radiofrequency devices have been developed and are presently being investigated for their effects on photorejuvenation.

More recently, a prototype in-home NAFL device for the treatment of solar lentigines has been developed (Laserscript; Palomar Medical). This 1410-nm, nonablative diode was used to treat 33 patients in a pilot trial in which subjects treated themselves with energies up to 30 mJ per microbeam for 4 weeks, and were followed for 3 months. At 1 month after the last treatment, two-thirds of blinded evaluators correctly identified the post-treatment image as "better" for 84% of the treated lesions.[46]

Home-based hair growth devices, such as the Hairmax Laser Comb (Lexington International, LLC, Boca Raton, FL, USA), Laser Cap (Transdermal Cap, Inc, Gates Mills, OH, USA), and TOPHAT655 device (Apira Science, Inc, Newport, CA, USA) incorporate a low-level light therapy concept also found in their in-office counterparts. These hair-growth devices contain low-powered laser diodes with wavelengths in the region of 630 to 670 nm, and are thought to induce proliferative activity in hair follicles resulting in terminalization of vellus human hair follicles. In a double-blind, randomized controlled trial of 41 males, the laser group received 25-minute treatments in a bicycle-helmet–like apparatus (TOPHAT655) every other day for 16 weeks. When hair counts at 16 weeks were compared with baseline counts, a 39% increase in hair was demonstrated ($P = .001$) in the laser-treated group.[47]

Several home-based hair-removal devices are available that attempt to replicate office devices, including the Tria Laser using a diode 810-nm laser (Tria Beauty, Inc, Dublin, CA, USA) and the Silk'n (Home Skinovations, Yokneam, Israel) that was developed according to the concept of IPL technology. To more safely treat Fitzpatrick skin types V and IV, a combined radiofrequency and IPL home device is presently being developed. Preliminary results show safety and efficacy. Similar to light-based in-office solutions, several home-based acne devices are also currently available. These devices use blue and red light diodes, heat, and IPL to treat mild to moderate acne, especially among patients who are hesitant to consider or have already failed other therapeutic options.

SUMMARY

With numerous innovations within cutaneous laser surgery, the future looks bright. In fact, in addition to perfecting already established treatment modalities, the scope of the field is continuously expanding, with new clinical indications being added to the armamentarium of laser experts. More selective treatment of existing targets ensures improved efficacy, with fewer side effects and treatment sessions. The identification of new targets allows for more effective treatment of common cutaneous conditions. Adjunctive applications, whether in drug delivery or identification of skin cancer, optimize treatment results and the diagnostic acumen of clinicians. There is no doubt that laser treatments are here to stay; the one exciting enquiry remaining, however, is what will appear next on the horizon.

REFERENCES

1. Srinivas CR, Kumaresan M. Lasers for vascular lesions: standard guidelines of care. Indian J Dermatol Venereol Leprol 2011;77(3):349–68.
2. Natalie K. Selective photothermolysis. Available at: http://plasticsurgery.about.com/od/glossary/g/selective_PTL.htm. Accessed August 09, 2012.
3. Gold MH, Goldman MP. 5-Aminolevulinic acid photodynamic therapy: where we have been and where we are going. Dermatol Surg 2004;30(8): 1077–84.
4. Divaris DX, Kennedy JC, Pottier RH. Phototoxic damage to sebaceous glands and hair follicles of mice after systemic administration of 5-aminolevulinic acid correlates with localized protoporphyrin IX fluorescence. Am J Pathol 1990;136(4):891–7.
5. Sakamoto FH, Lopes JD, Anderson RR. Photodynamic therapy for acne vulgaris: a critical review from basics to clinical practice: part I. Acne vulgaris: when and why consider photodynamic therapy? J Am Acad Dermatol 2010;63(2):183–94.
6. Gold MH, Bradshaw VL, Boring MM, et al. Treatment of sebaceous gland hyperplasia by photodynamic therapy with 5-aminolevulinic acid and a blue light source or intense pulsed light source. J Drugs Dermatol 2004;3(Suppl 6):S6–9.
7. Alster TS, Tanzi EL. Photodynamic therapy with topical aminolevulinic acid and pulsed dye laser irradiation for sebaceous hyperplasia. J Drugs Dermatol 2003;2(5):501–4.
8. Horfelt C, Funk J, Frohm-Nilsson M, et al. Topical methyl aminolaevulinate photodynamic therapy for treatment of facial acne vulgaris: results of a randomized, controlled study. Br J Dermatol 2006; 155(3):608–13.
9. Wiegell SR, Wulf HC. Photodynamic therapy of acne vulgaris using 5-aminolevulinic acid versus methyl aminolevulinate. J Am Acad Dermatol 2006;54(4): 647–51.
10. Wiegell SR, Wulf HC. Photodynamic therapy of acne vulgaris using methyl aminolaevulinate: a blinded,

randomized, controlled trial. Br J Dermatol 2006; 154(5):969–76.

11. Pollock B, Turner D, Stringer MR, et al. Topical aminolaevulinic acid-photodynamic therapy for the treatment of acne vulgaris: a study of clinical efficacy and mechanism of action. Br J Dermatol 2004;151(3):616–22.

12. Hongcharu W, Taylor CR, Chang Y, et al. Topical ALA-photodynamic therapy for the treatment of acne vulgaris. J Invest Dermatol 2000;115(2): 183–92.

13. Jeong E, Hong JW, Min JA, et al. Topical ALA-photodynamic therapy for acne can induce apoptosis of sebocytes and down-regulate their TLR-2 and TLR-4 expression. Ann Dermatol 2011; 23(1):23–32.

14. Sakamoto FH, Doukas AG, Farinelli WA, et al. Selective photothermolysis to target sebaceous glands: theoretical estimation of parameters and preliminary results using a free electron laser. Lasers Surg Med 2012;44(2):175–83.

15. Winstanley D, Blalock T, Houghton N, et al. Treatment of sebaceous hyperplasia with a novel 1,720-nm laser. J Drugs Dermatol 2012;11(11):1323–6.

16. Munavalli G. Single-center, prospective study on the efficacy and safety of micro-focused ultrasound with visualization for the non-invasive treatment of moderate to severe facial acne. Abstract presented at American Society for Laser Medicine and Surgery Conference. Boston, April 4–6, 2013.

17. Palm M, Massaki A, Fabi SG, et al. Laser lipolysis. In: Goldman MP, editor. Lasers and energy devices for the skin. 2nd edition. London: Informa Healthcare; 2012. p. 325–38.

18. Echague AV, Casas G, Rivera FP, et al. Over time histological tissue changes after non-invasive treatment with a 1210 nm laser. Abstract presented at American Society for Laser Medicine and Surgery Conference. Boston, April 4–6, 2013.

19. Centurion P, Noriega A. Fat preserving by laser 1210-nm. J Cosmet Laser Ther 2013;15(1):2–12.

20. Allemann I, Kaufman J. Fractional photothermolysis—an update. Lasers Med Sci 2010;25:137–44.

21. Jung JY, Cho SB, Chung HJ, et al. Treatment of periorbital wrinkles with 1550- and 1565-nm Er:glass fractional photothermolysis lasers: a simultaneous split-face trial. J Eur Acad Dermatol Venereol 2010; 25:811–8.

22. Ross EV, Miller L, Mishra V, et al. Clinical evaluation of a non-ablative 1940-nm fractional laser. Abstract presented at American Society for Laser Medicine and Surgery Conference. Boston, April 4–6, 2013.

23. Lee WR, Shen SC, Lai HH, et al. Transdermal drug delivery enhanced and controlled by erbium:YAG laser: a comparative study of lipophilic and hydrophilic drugs. J Control Release 2001;75:155–66.

24. Oni G, Brown SA, Kenkel JM. Can fractional lasers enhance transdermal absorption of topical lidocaine in an in vivo animal model? Lasers Surg Med 2012; 44:168–74.

25. Haedersdal M, Sakamoto FH, Farinelli WA, et al. Fractional CO(2) laser-assisted drug delivery. Lasers Surg Med 2010;42:113–22.

26. Gomez C, Costela A, Garcia-Moreno I, et al. Skin laser treatments enhancing trans- dermal delivery of ALA. J Pharm Sci 2011;100:223–31.

27. Waibel J, Wulkan A. Treatment of hypertrophic scars using laser assisted corticosteroids vs laser assisted 5-fluoruracil delivery. Abstract presented at American Society for Laser Medicine and Surgery Conference. Boston, April 4–6, 2013.

28. Oni G, Lequeux C, Cho MJ, et al. Transdermal delivery of adipocyte-derived stem cells using a fractional ablative laser. Aesthet Surg J 2013;33(1): 109–16.

29. Kotlus BS. Treatment of refractory axillary hyperhidrosis with a 1320-nm Nd:YAG laser. J Cosmet Laser Ther 2011;13(4):193–5.

30. Goldman A, Wollina U. Subdermal Nd-YAG laser for axillary hyperhidrosis. Dermatol Surg 2008;34(6): 756–62.

31. Yanes FD. G: laser-assisted minimally invasive surgery for primary hyperhidrosis. Abstract presented at American Society for Laser Medicine and Surgery Conference. Boston, April 4–6, 2013.

32. Bechara FG, Georgas D, Sand M, et al. Effects of a long-pulsed 800-nm diode laser on axillary hyperhidrosis: a randomized controlled half-side comparison study. Dermatol Surg 2012;38(5):736–40.

33. Johnson JE, O'Shaughnessy KF, Kim S. Microwave thermolysis of sweat glands. Lasers Surg Med 2012;44(1):20–5.

34. Glaser DA, Coleman WP 3rd, Fan LK, et al. A randomized, blinded clinical evaluation of a novel microwave device for treating axillary hyperhidrosis: the dermatologic reduction in underarm perspiration study. Dermatol Surg 2012;38(2):185–91.

35. Nestor M, Hyunhee P. Randomized, double-blind, controlled pilot study of the efficacy and safety of micro-focused ultrasound for the treatment of axillary hyperhidrosis. Abstract presented at American Society for Laser Medicine and Surgery Conference. Boston, April 4–6, 2013.

36. Huang N, Jiang F, Chen D, et al. Photothermal effect of single-walled carbon nano-horns. Abstract presented at American Society for Laser Medicine and Surgery Conference. Boston, April 4–6, 2013.

37. Bahmani B, Anvari B. Targeted photodestruction of ovarian cancer cells using Anti-HER2 conjugated ICG-loaded polymeric nanoparticles. Abstract presented at American Society for Laser Medicine and Surgery Conference. Boston, April 4–6, 2013.

38. Benito M, Martín V, Blanco MD, et al. Cooperative effect of 5-aminolevulinic acid and gold nanoparticles for photodynamic therapy of cancer. J Pharm Sci 2013. http://dx.doi.org/10.1002/jps.23621.

39. Lui H, Zhao J, McLean D, et al. Real-time Raman spectroscopy for in vivo skin cancer diagnosis. Cancer Res 2012;72(10):2491–500.

40. Sierra R, Mirkov M. Impact of pulse duration from nanoseconds to picoseconds on the thermal and mechanical effects during laser interaction with tattoo targets. Abstract presented at American Society for Laser Medicine and Surgery Conference. Boston, April 4–6, 2013.

41. Saedi N, Metelitsa A, Petrell K, et al. Treatment of tattoos with a picosecond alexandrite laser: a prospective trial. Arch Dermatol 2012;148(12):1360–3.

42. Brauer JA, Reddy KK, Anolik R, et al. Successful and rapid treatment of blue and green tattoo pigment with a novel picosecond laser. Arch Dermatol 2012;148(7):820–3.

43. Brauer J, Correa L, Bernstein L, et al. Evaluation of a picosecond 755nm alexandrite laser and defractive lens array for scarring. Abstract presented at American Society for Laser Medicine and Surgery Conference. Boston, April 4–6, 2013.

44. Brauer J, Correa L, Bernstein L, et al. We're not stretching the truth: treatment of striae with a picosecond 755nm alexandrite laser and defractive lens array. Abstract presented at American Society for Laser Medicine and Surgery Conference. Boston, April 4–6, 2013.

45. Metelitsa AI, Green JB. Home-use laser and light devices for the skin: an update. Semin Cutan Med Surg 2011;30(3):144–7.

46. Weiss R, Doherty S. Clinical study of physician-directed home-use non-ablative fractional device for the treatment of pigmented lesions. Abstract presented at American Society for Laser Medicine and Surgery Conference. Boston, April 4–6, 2013.

47. Lanzafame R, Blanche R, Bodian A, et al. The growth of human scalp hair mediated by visible red light laser and LED sources in males. Abstract presented at American Society for Laser Medicine and Surgery Conference. Boston, April 4–6, 2013.

Ultrasound Skin Tightening

Kira Minkis, MD, PhD[a], Murad Alam, MD, MSCI[a,b,c],*

KEYWORDS

- Skin tightening • Skin lifting • Photo-rejuvenation • Ultrasound • Photoaging

KEY POINTS

- Skin laxity is a common sign of photoaging.
- Skin lifting and tightening is a desirable outcome by a most patients interesting in photorejuvenation.
- Noninvasive treatment options for skin tightening and skin lifting are limited.
- Intense focused ultrasound has been shown to provide skin lifting and tightening, making it the only device approved by the Food and Drug Administration for this indication.
- Ultrasound is a safe and efficacious treatment for mild skin tightening and lifting.

INTRODUCTION

Photoaging of the face occurs in a semipredictable stepwise progression that includes both textural and pigmentary alterations to the skin. In the initial steps of skin aging, dynamic rhytides are evident in areas of skin movement; these eventuate into static rhytides. With further age, the skin, both facial as well as areas off the face, begin to develop laxity, which is often most evident in the jowls and submental skin. Photorejuvenation of the skin, in its optimum, should therefore address all of these components of the aging skin. Traditionally, various energy-delivery devices were used to treat several components of skin aging, including rhytides, laxity, and dyschromia, such as ablative carbon dioxide or erbium:yttrium-aluminum-garnet devices, as well as treatments such as deep chemical peels and dermabrasion. These methods relied on ablation of the epidermis causing reepithelialization while delivering significant thermal injury to the dermis sufficient to stimulate a robust wound-healing response with subsequent collagen remodeling and contraction leading to decreased rhytides, improvement in skin texture, skin tightening, and improvement in pigmentation. However, despite significant improvement in these skin characteristics and efficacy of these treatments, significant patient downtime, long and painful posttreatment healing, and substantial side effects were major drawbacks of these ablative procedures.

In recent years, multiple different treatment modalities have become available for treatment of skin wrinkling and laxity in a nonablative manner. These include lasers and light devices, infrared energy devices, and energy-based procedures, including radiofrequency ablation. These allow the use of thermal energy to target the reticular dermis and subcutis in an effort to cause tissue contraction and dermal remodeling while minimizing undesirable epidermal injury. As a result, "downtime" is minimized with expedient postprocedure healing, allowing for the patient to proceed with regular activities shortly after treatment, minimizing the necessity to interrupt a busy patient's work or social schedule. Additionally, minimal epidermal injury allows for safer

Funding Sources: No funding provided.

Conflict of Interest: The authors report no conflicts of interest.

[a] Department of Dermatology, Northwestern University, 676 North St Clair Street, Suite 1600, Chicago, IL 60611, USA; [b] Department of Otolaryngology-Head and Neck Surgery, Northwestern University, 676 North St Clair Street, Suite 1600, Chicago, IL 60611, USA; [c] Department of Surgery, Northwestern University, 676 North St Clair Street, Suite 1600, Chicago, IL 60611, USA
* Corresponding author. Department of Dermatology, Northwestern University, 676 North St Clair Street, Suite 1600, Chicago, IL 60611.
E-mail address: m-alam@northwestern.edu

Dermatol Clin 32 (2014) 71–77
http://dx.doi.org/10.1016/j.det.2013.09.001
0733-8635/14/$ – see front matter © 2014 Elsevier Inc. All rights reserved.

treatment among a wider range of skin types and reduces the risk of adverse events compared with either ablative resurfacing or more invasive surgical procedures, such as rhytidectomy. However, the drawback of these safer nonablative methods are that, relative to their invasive and ablative counterparts, the results are often modest, less reliable, and inconsistent duration of benefit. Individual variation in responsiveness to noninvasive skin tightening has also been significant. Ultrasound is an energy modality that can be focused and penetrates deeper in the tissue to cause thermal coagulation. Intense focused ultrasound (IFUS) for skin rejuvenation has been shown in recent studies to be safe and effective for skin tightening and lifting.

Ulthera System (Ulthera Inc, Mesa, AZ) is an IFUS device that delivers inducible energy to selected foci within the dermis and subcutis leading to the generation of heat and selective coagulative changes. The generated heat causes initiation of the tissue repair cascade in which the end result is a tightening effect of the skin. Results from several studies have led Ulthera to receive the first and only Food and Drug Administration approval for skin lifting, initially for eyebrow lifting in 2009, followed several years later with an approval for skin lifting of the neck and submentum. A unique added advantage to the use of ultrasound for skin rejuvenation is the direct visualization of the dermis and subcutaneous structures before treatment, which adds an extra level of safety to the treatment. Unfocused ultrasound energy can be used to image the treatment area while focused ultrasound energy can induce thermal injury of the mid to deep reticular dermis without damaging more superficial layers. Direct visualization allows for the identification of key anatomic structures and their depths and adapting the energy deposition to deliberate and precise locations in the dermis or subcutis. The device is particularly efficacious for treatment of patients with moderate laxity of the skin on the face for "lifting" of the eyebrow, neck, and submentum; however, recently it also has been used in various other locations and applications, including tightening of the skin of the buttock, décolleté, and other locations on the face, as well as for the treatment of acne and hyperhidrosis.

DEVICE PROPERTIES/TECHNOLOGY

Ultrasound is the sound wave frequencies above the range of human hearing (18–20 kHz). Ulthera operates at 4 to 7 MHz. The ultrasound imaging is adapted to the visualization of the first 8 mm of tissue, thus specifically allowing for imaging of skin. The dual-modality ultrasound combines the capability of real-time imaging allowing visualizing below the skin's surface and providing precisely placed "thermal coagulation points" (TCPs) at prescribed depths. This creates small micro-coagulation zones of 1 mm^3 to 1.5 mm^3, which cause thermal contraction of tissue. The subsequent wound-healing response results in collagen stimulation.

Ulthera Device

The Ulthera device consists of a central power unit, a computer, and interchangeable delivery handpieces. The same handpiece contains a transducer that enables sequential imaging (lower-energy ultrasound, allowing visualization of dermal and subcutaneous structures) and treatment (delivery of higher-energy ultrasound exposures). Multiple source settings can be controlled, including power output, exposure time, length of exposure line, distance between exposure zones, and time delay after each exposure.

The device initially had 3 handpieces:

1. Superficial: 7.5 MHz, 3.0-mm focus depth
2. Intermediate: 7.5 MHz, 4.5-mm focus depth
3. Deep: 4.4 MHz, 4.5-mm focus depth

Most recently, a 19-MHz transducer capable of producing focal TCPs at depths of 1.5 mm into the dermis was introduced to cause more superficial dermal neocollagenesis.

Human cadaveric tissues have demonstrated that penetration depth is determined by frequency, such that higher-frequency waves produce a shallow focal injury zone and lower-frequency waves have a greater depth of penetration to produce TCPs at deeper layers.[1]

Each probe delivers the energy in a straight 25-mm line with TCPs 0.5 to 5.0 mm apart at a given depth within the tissue. Short pulse durations (25–50 ms) and relatively low energy (in the 0.4–1.2 J range), depending on the particular transducer, confine the TCPs to their target depth. The handpiece moves in a straight line at the set conditions (power, duration) and at the selective variables (length of treatment, spacing of exposures) to produce uniform tissue exposures for each "line" of IFUS treatment. Human cadaveric studies, as well as preclinical studies in porcine skin and prerhytidectomy excision skin have confirmed consistency in the depth, size, and orientation of TCP created by IFUS, in the subdermal soft tissue and deeper superficial musculoaponeurotic system (SMAS) layers, while preserving immediately adjacent soft tissue and structures.[2–5]

The thermal injury is confined by keeping the pulse duration relatively short. Providing the energy delivered is not excessive for the given focal depth and frequency emitted by a given transducer, the epidermal surface remains unaffected. Therefore, the need for epidermal cooling is eliminated.[3,4] Because the tissue is altered by arrays of small zones of focal damage rather than ablation of an entire macroscopic area, rapid healing occurs from tissue immediately adjacent to the thermal lesions. This is somewhat analogous to fractional laser ablation, except IFUS affects only the deep dermal and subcutaneous tissue.

The tightening effect of ultrasound treatment is based on coagulative heating of specific zones of the dermis and subcutaneous tissue. The ultrasound energy is focused, such that thermal coagulation occurs only where the sound waves meet at discrete separated TCPs. The size of the points varies based on the specific frequency and power settings used. This eventuates into nonsurgical tissue lifting without affecting the surface of the skin. Apart from ionizing radiation, ultrasound is the only type of inducible energy that can be delivered arbitrarily deeply into tissue in a selective manner. The treatment is programmable for various depths and spacing based on transducer selection with the variability of energy delivery in the actual treatment occurring only secondary to improper skin contact when the transducer is applied on the skin. For the more superficial treatment depth, the spacing between TCPs is closer. To avoid surface effect, less energy is applied when using the more superficial delivery of energy.

MECHANISM

Transcutaneous application of ultrasound into whole-organ soft tissue produces coagulative necrosis resulting primarily from thermal mechanisms.[1,6,7] The ultrasound field vibrates tissue, creating friction between molecules, which absorb mechanical energy that leads to secondary generation of heat. Selective coagulative change is affected within the focal region of the beam, with the immediately adjacent tissue spared.[2–5]

In IFUS, energy is deposited in short pulses in the millisecond domain (50–200 ms). Avoiding cavitational processes, a frequency in the megahertz (MHz) domain is used with energy levels deposited at each treatment site being on the order of 0.5 to 10 J. It is estimated that the device heats tissue to 65°C to 75°C, the critical temperature at which collagen denaturation occurs with instigation of the tissue repair cascade. Precise microcoagulation zones deep in the dermis, as well as the superficial musculoaponeurotic

system, have been demonstrated.[3,6] Suh and colleagues[8] demonstrated histologic evidence that both dermal collagen and elastic fibers were significantly regenerated and increased in number, resulting in thickening of the reticular dermis with no significant change in the epidermis. The investigators concluded that it is via this dermal collagen regeneration that the rejuvenation of infraorbital laxity is achieved.

This microcoagulation is thought to cause gradual tightening of the skin through collagen contraction and remodeling. The onset of collagen denaturation with subsequent tissue contraction by 3 months, and the duration of clinical lifting responses lasting for about 1 year are similar to treatment with radiofrequency, ultrasonography, or laser energy sources.

INDICATIONS/APPLICATIONS

Results from several studies have lead Ulthera to receive the first and only Food and Drug Administration approval for skin lift, initially for eyebrow lifting in 2009, followed several years later with an approval for skin lifting of the neck and submentum. However, the applicability and indications have expanded in recent years with a multitude of studies exploring off-label use for skin tightening, as well as applying IFUS for treatment of other skin diseases.

The first clinical study in noncadaveric skin was performed by Alam and colleagues.[9] Thirty-five subjects were treated and evaluated for safety and efficacy of treatment. The investigators found 86% of the subjects achieved significant improvement 90 days after treatment as measured by blinded physician assessment. Photographic measurements demonstrated a mean brow lift of 1.7 mm at 90 days.

Chan and colleagues[10] evaluated the safety of IFUS on skin tightening in 49 Chinese subjects. All of the treated subjects underwent full-facial and neck treatment with no oral analgesia or topical anesthetics. The investigators reported more than half of the treated subjects rated pain as severe and experienced only minor, transient adverse effects.

Suh and colleagues[11] evaluated 22 Korean subjects (Fitzpatrick skin types III–VI) after full-face treatment.

- All treated subjects reported an improvement with 91% demonstrating improvement in objective score values at the nasolabial fold and jaw line. The average objective score of nasolabial fold and jaw line improvement was 1.91 (rated on a subjective scale where 1 = improved and 2 = much improved).

- Subjectively, 77% of the subjects reported much improvement of nasolabial folds, and 73% reported much improvement of the jaw line. The average subjective scores of nasolabial fold and jaw line improvement were 1.77 and 1.72, respectively.

Skin biopsies obtained from 11 subjects at baseline and 2 months after treatment confirmed an increase in reticular dermal collagen and dermal thickening, with elastic fibers appearing more parallel and straighter than pretreatment specimens.

Lee and colleagues[12] evaluated multipass IFUSs in a study in which 10 subjects were treated on the face and neck with the 4-MHz, 4.5-mm probe first, followed by the 7-MHz, 3.0-mm probe. The investigators reported an 80% improvement by blinded physician assessment and 90% reported subjective improvement 90 days after treatment.

Suh and colleagues[8] treated 15 subjects with a single pass to the lower infraorbital region with a 7-MHz 3-mm transducer and demonstrated objective improvement in all study subjects and subjective improvement in most (86%) of the subjects treated.

Alster and Tanzi[13] first reported the efficacy of IFUS on body sites. Eighteen study subjects were evaluated using paired areas on the arms, knees, and medial thighs where dual-plane treatment with the 4-MHz 4.5-mm-depth and 7-MHz 3-mm-depth transducer was compared with single-plane treatment with the 4-MHz 4.5-mm-depth transducer alone. Global assessment scores of skin tightening and lifting were determined by 2 blinded physician raters and graded using a quartile grading scale. At the 6-month follow-up visit, significant improvement was seen in all treated areas, with the upper arms and knees demonstrating more skin lifting and tightening than the thighs. Areas receiving dual-plane treatment had slightly better clinical scores than those receiving a single-plane treatment in all 3 sites, potentially secondary to more superficial dermal collagen remodeling. The investigators also demonstrated high patient satisfaction, reporting 13 of the 16 patients were "highly satisfied" with the procedure and opted to undergo similar focused ultrasound treatment of different facial and body areas after the conclusion of the study.

Sasaki and Tevez[14] studied efficacy of IFUS for multiple indications. Using the new 19-MHz 1.5-mm superficial transducer, they treated 19 subjects in the periorbital region with 45 lines on each side, and an additional 45 lines using the 7-MHz 3-mm as the second depth over the orbital rim. A single treatment produced an average elevation between 1 and 2 mm (7%–8% increase from baseline) in each of the 19 subjects. Periorbital skin tightening was rated as moderate between a 3-month and 6-month period. Beneficial effects were noted as early as 6 weeks (particularly eyelid and periorbital skin) but most subjects appreciated a smoothing and tightening effect between 3 and 6 months. Observed responses lasted about 6 months to 1.5 years. Body sites treated in this study included brachium (44), periumbilicus (6), décolletage (5), knee (4), buttocks (2), inner thigh (1), and hand (1). Treatment protocols varied according to skin thickness at the treated location. Blinded evaluator assessment scores revealed moderate improvement in the periorbital area, inner brachium, periumbilicus, and knees. Improvement was less consistent in the inner thighs, décolletage, hands, and buttocks.

In a larger series of pilot studies and clinical investigations, which in total included 197 patients, Sasaki and Tevez[15] compared horizontal and vertical vectors in the brow and marionette regions while maintaining constant depth and energy. Vertical vectors produced significant lifting over horizontally placed treatment lines. The investigators also showed that significantly greater lifting was achieved at sites with more treatment lines and higher joule energy.

Recently reported studies and presentations at scientific meetings have demonstrated the growing number of investigations under way evaluating the applicability of IFUS for a multitude of treatment sites as well as expanding list of indications. Data also have been presented supporting the use of IFUS for wrinkling around the knee,[16] tightening of the neck,[17] tightening of the décolletage,[18] and lifting of the buttock.[19] Additionally, IFUS is being explored for the treatment of axillary hyperhidrosis[20] and acne. Successful treatment of silicone lip deformity using IFUS also has been described.[21] The same group also used IFUS to control edema and shape the nasal skin after rhinoplasty.[22]

PATIENT SELECTION

Patients who would be good candidates are those wishing to avoid surgical facelift but would like treatment of skin laxity. The ideal patient for nonsurgical tissue tightening displays mild to moderate skin and soft tissue laxity. Preferably, patients should be nonsmokers and not obese and ideal candidates should not have major sagging or excessive photoaging, as their ability to create collagen in response to thermal injury may be inadequate.

Additionally, younger patients would be better suited for the thermal energy treatment, as they should possess collagen fibers of optimal quantity and size as well as the most advantageous fiber orientation to allow maximal thermal absorption. Moreover, younger patients tend to have a more robust wound-healing response. Severe aging, tissue heaviness, and fullness would also negatively impact results, as it may impede the lifting effects after thermally induced collagen shortening.

IFUS is safe across all skin types. Suh and colleagues[11] was the first to demonstrate safety and efficacy of IFUS in Asian skin (Fitzpatrick skin type III–VI). The few absolute contraindications include active infection or open skin at the treatment site, cystic acne, and pregnancy. Relative contraindications include medical conditions and/or medications that alter or impair wound healing.

Of paramount importance before treatment is setting realistic expectations for patients. A patient with unrealistic expectations of treatment would be a relative contraindication to treatment, as the clinical improvements are often subtle, with most studies demonstrating mild to moderate improvement, unlike that of surgical treatment options. It is helpful to have good photography obtained before and following treatment, as well as a detailed discussion of expected results, limitations, and potential for no appreciable clinical improvement.

TECHNIQUE/TREATMENT PROTOCOL
General

The depth of treatment, and therefore probe to use for a specific area, is dictated by the thickness of the skin at the treatment site, such that areas of thinnest skin (ie, neck and periocular area) should be treated with superficial depth probes, whereas cheeks and submentum should be treated with deepest depth probes followed by additional treatment with a superficial probe. Initial treatments had lower density of lines placed at just one depth.

There has been a growing trend toward the targeting of multiple depths of TCPs to affect collagen at multiple treatment planes for enhancing the efficacy of treatment.[13–15] With dual-depth treatment, with the deeper plane treated first, a higher concentration of treatment lines can be delivered in uniform matrices in the targeted anatomy.

Topical skin care products, such as topical retinoids and alpha and beta hydroxyacids, should be discontinued about 2 weeks before treatment. Patients should be advised not to apply facial creams, lotions, powders, and foundations on the treatment day. All metal facial jewelry should be removed. Patients with a history of viral infections should be placed on prophylactic antivirals 2 days before and 6 days after the procedure. Before treatment, the skin is cleaned of any facial products, makeup, or sunscreen. Each treatment region is outlined with a planning card to determine the number of treatment columns. Next, ultrasound gel is applied to the target site, and the selected transducer is placed firmly on the skin and activated, taking care to ensure that the entire transducer is evenly coupled to the skin surface. The ultrasound gel may need to be reapplied frequently to ensure proper tissue imaging and coupling. The correct placement of the ultrasound probe is confirmed on the screen as acoustic coupling can be visualized on the ultrasound images. Focal depth also can be visualized on the monitor in the ultrasound image and depending on the probe used and targeted site, this can be lined up with the corresponding layer of the deep dermis to SMAS. A parallel linear array of ultrasound pulses is manually delivered with minimal spacing. The total number of lines placed in a treatment area will depend on the size of the treatment area and particular parameters chosen with up to 600 to 800 lines of ultrasound pulses for a full face treatment. Caution should be exercised (and treatment avoided) over soft tissue augmentation material and implants, over the thyroid gland, and inside the orbital rim (currently, there are no commercially available eye shields that have been shown to effectively block ultrasound energy). Following completion of treatment, the ultrasound gel is removed and an emollient cream applied. Patients may return immediately to their usual activities. Medical skin care regimens can be resumed within 1 week.

Pain

Individual published reports of pain in response to the treatment range from mild to severe. Sufficient pain management is important to affect the overall treatment experience for the patient. The specific type of pain control varies based on physician preference. MacGregor and Tanzi[23] report using a combination of oral anxiolytics (5–10 mg of diazepam) and intramuscular narcotics (50–75 mg meperidine) 20 to 30 minutes before treatment to alleviate discomfort in most patients. Other investigators have described a variety of methods of pain control, including use of high-dose nonsteroidal anti-inflammatory drugs, narcotics (oral or intravenous), anesthetics (topical or local injection), conscious sedation, distracting massages, and cold techniques.[24] Logically, the higher energy and deeper probe is associated with increased pain. According to Sasaki and Tevez,[15] the most patients who received treatment to the midface and neck did not require a local nerve block or lidocaine, whereas patients treated on the forehead/brow may require local anesthesia or nerve blocks because of the thinness of tissues overlying the frontal bone. Moderate to significant intraoperative pain was experienced most commonly to the décolletage, brachium, knee, and periumbilical sites.[14]

Safety

In general, IFUS has a good side-effect profile, with most side effects being temporary. Side effects include minimal pain, transient erythema, edema, and purpura, which are typically minimal and not persistent. Uncommonly, striated linear skin patterns occur and spontaneously resolve within a few weeks but also can be treated with high-potency topical steroids.

The most concerning complication in the immediate posttreatment period of IFUS is motor nerve paresis. This complication is limited to case reports.[23] The areas at the greatest risk for injury are locations in which the branches of the facial nerve take on a superficial course, namely the temporal branch of the trigeminal nerve at the temple as well as the marginal mandibular nerve at the jawline. Symptoms typically occur within the first 1 to 12 hours posttreatment, likely secondary to nerve inflammation. Complete resolution is expected in 2 to 6 weeks.[23] In patients who notice facial muscle twitching during treatment, the area should be iced immediately and consideration given to an anti-inflammatory medication. Sasaki and Tevez[15] reported 3 patients who developed transient dysesthesia (numbness or hypersensitivity) to the deep branch of the supraorbital nerve that lasted for 3 to 7 days, and 4 patients developed numbness along the mandible after treatment on the cheeks that resolved without sequelae 2 to 3 weeks after IFUS treatment.[15]

SUMMARY

IFUS delivers ultrasound energy to predetermined depths in the deep dermis and subdermal tissue, creating TCPs that cause subsequent neocollagenesis and tissue contraction, which leads to lifting and tightening of the skin over the ensuing months posttreatment. As the energy delivery is precisely focused, deeper and more superficial, as well as immediately adjacent, tissue is spared, contributing to a very good safety profile and allowing treatment of dark skin phototypes. Clinical parameters of treatment are always evolving to maximize effectiveness of treatment. Likewise, indications of treatments have expanded vastly to include nonfacial skin tightening and experimental treatment of other dermatologic conditions, as well as treatments in various other medical fields.

REFERENCES

1. White WM, Laubach HJ, Makin IR, et al. Selective transcutaneous delivery of energy to facial subdermal tissues using the ultrasound therapy system [abstract]. Lasers Surg Med 2006;38(Suppl 18):113.
2. White WM, Makin IR, Slayton MH, et al. Selective transcutaneous delivery of energy to porcine soft tissues using intense ultrasound (IUS). Lasers Surg Med 2008;40:67–75.
3. White WM, Makin IR, Barthe PG, et al. Selective creation of thermal injury zones in the superficial musculoaponeurotic system using intense ultrasound therapy: a new target for noninvasive facial rejuvenation. Arch Facial Plast Surg 2007;9:22–9.
4. Laubach HJ, Makin IR, Barthe PG, et al. Intense focused ultrasound: evaluation of a new treatment modality for precise microcoagulation within the skin. Dermatol Surg 2008;34:727–34.
5. Gliklich RE, White WM, Slayton MH, et al. Clinical pilot study of intense ultrasound therapy to deep dermal facial skin and subcutaneous tissues. Arch Facial Plast Surg 2007;9:88–95.
6. Laubach HJ, Barthe PG, Makin IRS, et al. Confined thermal damage with intense ultrasound (IUS) [abstract]. Lasers Surg Med 2006;38(Suppl 18):32.
7. Makin IR, Mast TD, Faidi W, et al. Miniaturized ultrasound arrays for interstitial ablation and imaging. Ultrasound Med Biol 2005;31:1539–50.
8. Suh DH, Oh YJ, Lee SJ, et al. Intense focused ultrasound tightening for the treatment of infraorbital laxity. J Cosmet Laser Ther 2012;14:290–5.
9. Alam M, White LE, Martin N, et al. Ultrasound tightening of facial and neck skin: a rater-blinded prospective cohort study. J Am Acad Dermatol 2010; 62:262–9.
10. Chan NP, Shek SY, Yu CS, et al. Safety study of transcutaneous focused ultrasound for noninvasive skin tightening in Asians. Lasers Surg Med 2011;43:366–75.
11. Suh DH, Shin MK, Lee SJ, et al. Intense focused ultrasound tightening in Asian skin: clinical and pathologic results. Dermatol Surg 2011;37:1595–602.
12. Lee HS, Jang WS, Cha YJ, et al. Multiple pass ultrasound tightening of skin laxity of the lower face and neck. Dermatol Surg 2012;38:20–7.
13. Alster TS, Tanzi EL. Noninvasive lifting of arm, thigh, and knee skin with transcutaneous intense focused ultrasound. Dermatol Surg 2012;38:754–9.
14. Sasaki GH, Tevez A. Microfocused ultrasound for nonablative skin and subdermal tightening to the periorbitum and body sites: preliminary report on

eighty-two patients. J Chem Dermatol Sci Appl 2012;2:108–16.

15. Sasaki GH, Tevez A. Clinical efficacy and safety of focused-image ultrasonography: a 2-year experience. Aesthet Surg J 2012;32:601–12.

16. Gold MH. Ulthera—A single center, prospective study on the efficacy of the micro-focused ultrasound for the non-invasive treatment of skin wrinkles above the knee. Data presented at the American Society for Dermatologic Surgery Meeting. Atlanta, GA, October 11–14, 2012.

17. Elm KD, Schram SE, Wallander ID, et al. Evaluation of a high intensity focused ultrasound system for lifting and tightening of the neck. Data presented at the American Society for Dermatologic Surgery Meeting. Atlanta, GA, October 11–14, 2012.

18. Fabi SG, Massaki A, Goldman M. Evaluation of the micro-focused ultrasound system for lifting and tightening of the décolletage. Data presented at the American Society for Dermatologic Surgery Meeting. Atlanta, GA, October 11–14, 2012.

19. Goldberg D, Al-Dujaili Z. Micro-focused ultrasound for lifting and tightening skin laxity of the buttock. Data presented at the American Society for Dermatologic Surgery Meeting. Atlanta, GA, October 11–14, 2012.

20. Nestor MS. Micro-focused ultrasound for the treatment of axillary hyperhidrosis. Data Presented at the American Society for Dermatologic Surgery Meeting. Atlanta, GA, October 11–14, 2012.

21. Kornstein AN. Ulthera for silicone lip correction. Plast Reconstr Surg 2012;129(6):1014e–5e.

22. Kornstein AN. Ultherapy shrinks nasal skin after rhinoplasty following failure of conservative measures. Plast Reconstr Surg 2013;131(4):664e–6e.

23. MacGregor JL, Tanzi EL. Microfocused ultrasound for skin tightening. Semin Cutan Med Surg 2013;32:18–25.

24. Brobst RW, Ferguson M, Perkins SW. Ulthera: initial and six month results. Facial Plast Surg Clin North Am 2012;20:163–76.

Radiofrequency in Cosmetic Dermatology

Karen L. Beasley, MD*, Robert A. Weiss, MD

KEYWORDS

- Radiofrequency • Skin tightening • Body contouring • Cellulite reduction • Noninvasive
- Monopolar • Unipolar

KEY POINTS

- Radiofrequency (RF) has become an important and frequently used technology in cosmetic dermatology.
- RF is most commonly used for tissue heating and tightening as well as body contouring and cellulite reduction.
- RF treatments are safe, effective, and have minimal to no downtime.
- RF energy can be delivered by monopolar, bipolar, unipolar methods and can be combined with other light or energy sources.
- Continued research of RF devices will help to improve the efficacy and increase the knowledge about this rapidly developing technology.

INTRODUCTION

The demand for noninvasive methods of facial and body rejuvenation has experienced exponential growth over the last decade. There is a particular interest in safe and effective ways to decrease skin laxity and smooth irregular body contours and texture without downtime. These noninvasive treatments are being sought after because less time for recovery means less time lost from work and social endeavors. Radiofrequency (RF) treatments are traditionally titrated to be nonablative and are optimal for those wishing to avoid recovery time. Not only is there minimal recovery but there is also a high level of safety with aesthetic RF treatments.

RF energy has been used for decades in a variety of medical applications, including tissue electrodessication, cardiac catheter ablation, and endovenous ablation of varicose veins.[1,2] Unlike laser energy, RF energy does not depend on selective photothermolysis but rather heating of water;

therefore, any skin type may be treated. The mechanism of action of RF in a medical application is based on an oscillating electrical current forcing collisions between charged molecules and ions, which are then transformed into heat. RF-generated tissue heating has different biologic and clinical effects, depending on the depth of tissue targeted, the frequency used, and specific cooling of the dermis and epidermis. The depth of penetration of RF energy is inversely proportional to the frequency. Consequently, lower frequencies of RF are able to penetrate more deeply. RF technology also has the ability to noninvasively and selectively heat large volumes of subcutaneous adipose tissue. By selecting the appropriate electric field, one can obtain greater heating of fat or water.

In cosmetic dermatology, RF is most commonly used to noninvasively tighten lax skin; to contour the body by influencing adipocytes; and, consequently, to improve the appearance of cellulite. As a noninvasive treatment of facial rejuvenation

The Maryland Laser, Skin, and Vein Institute, 54 Scott Adam Road, Hunt Valley, MD 21030, USA
* Corresponding author. The Maryland Laser, Skin, and Vein Institute, 54 Scott Adam Road, Suite 301, Hunt Valley, MD 21030.
E-mail address: kbeasley@mdlsv.com

Dermatol Clin 32 (2014) 79–90
http://dx.doi.org/10.1016/j.det.2013.09.010

derm.theclinics.com

and skin tightening, the use of RF is typically reserved for deeper skin heating without causing ablation of the epidermis and dermis. RF devices are within the frequency range of 3 KHz to 24 GHz, which comprises an RF band, which is reserved for industrial, scientific, and medical (ISM) uses. The general population is most familiar with ISM bands for Wi-Fi 2.5- to 5.0-GHz radio bands used in the industrial sector. In clinical studies of lax skin treated with RF, the dermis, which is composed of collagen, elastin, and ground substances, has shown an immediate and temporary change in the helical structure of collagen. Electron microscopy from treated skin has revealed collagen fibrils with greater diameter compared with fibers pretreatment. Also, there was an increase in collagen expression as measured using Northern blot analysis.[3] It is also thought that RF thermal stimulation results in a microinflammatory stimulation of fibroblasts, which produces new collagen (neocollagenesis), new elastin (neoelastogenesis), and other substances to enhance dermal structure.[4] RF has not only been proven effective for skin tightening but it has also been studied and proven effective in diminishing adipocytes.

Body consciousness continues to increase as does the portion size and daily caloric count in our society. As the accessibility of food calories increases in all developed countries, so do the methods of reducing the effects of fat accumulation. Multiple modalities to induce adipocyte apoptosis in order to reduce pockets of fat noninvasively have recently become obtainable. These modalities primarily aim at targeting the properties of fat, which differentiate it from skin and muscle, thus resulting in selective removal or dissolution of fat otherwise known as lipolysis. By manipulating skin cooling, RF can be used for heating and reduction of fat. RF thermal stimulation of adipose tissue is thought to result in a thermal-mediated stimulation of adipocyte metabolism and augmented activity of lipase-mediated enzymatic degradation of triglycerides into free fatty acids and glycerol. Induction of apoptosis of fat cells is another proven mechanism.[5] In addition to fat reduction, RF can be used to improve the appearance of cellulite. Cellulite, the dimpled appearance of the skin caused by fatty deposits trapped and tethered between fibrous septa of the dermis, continues to be an elusive and highly sought after treatment. RF energy is able to heat the deep dermis and adipose tissue; hence, it should theoretically improve the cellulitic appearance of the skin.

RF can be delivered using monopolar, bipolar, or unipolar devices. Other variants of RF delivery include fractional, sublative, and combination technologies that add light, laser, massage, or electromagnetic fields (**Table 1**). There is also a novel multipolar RF device that delivers a field of energy to the skin and fat without contacting the skin. This article reviews the methods of RF delivery and highlights some of the most commonly used RF devices in cosmetic dermatology.

METHODS OF RF DELIVERY
Monopolar

The ISM bands were first established at the International Telecommunications Conference of the International Telecommunication Union in Atlantic City in 1947. The initial use of RF for medicine included the pinpoint coagulation of blood vessels during surgery. This use was the first use of monopolar RF requiring patients to have a grounding plate in contact with the skin. RF-induced heat ablation has been applied to other fields of dermatology, including soft tissue (basal cell carcinoma) ablation, endovenous ablation of saphenous system varicosities, and treatment of vascular abnormalities. There are many medical devices on the market, and each has wide-ranging methods of RF delivery. RF devices may be monopolar in which patients are grounded and the RF is delivered through the skin, into the body, and ultimately to the grounding electrode. Typically, RF travels through structures with the highest water content with greatest resistance by fat. In general, monopolar devices have a more deeply penetrating effect than bipolar or unipolar devices. Pain during the treatment is related to the duration of the pulse. Some devices are painful and some feel more like a heated massage. Monopolar RF can be delivered in a static or a dynamic fashion.

Monopolar devices may be delivered in a static or stamped mode in which a short 1- to 2-second cycle is delivered while the handpiece is held in place (Thermage, Solta Medical, Hayward, CA). Alternatively, monopolar RF may be delivered in a dynamic or a continuous pulse with constant rotation of the handpiece (Exilis, BTL, Prague, Czech Republic). In the static, stamped method, a single pulse is delivered; the handpiece is then moved to an adjacent marked area and fired again. This technique is performed for hundreds of pulses until a premarked area is treated. Each pulse is measured for temperature while spray cooling is applied so that a skin temperature of 45°C is not exceeded. With dynamic monopolar RF, the handpiece is continuously moved and specific areas of laxity can be targeted in a relatively short time to a final temperature that is monitored by continuous surface temperature measurements, often built into the handpiece. The dynamic devices are quicker but require more technique and skill, whereas the stamped devices are more tedious, take longer, but are easier to perform.

Bipolar

Other methods of RF delivery include bipolar, in which the RF travels from the positive to the negative pole, which is typically between 2 poles built into the handpiece. With a specific distance between the electrodes, the depth of penetration and heating is predetermined by the spacing of the electrodes and is typically confined to within 1 to 4 mm of the skin surface. It is commonly stated that the depth of penetration is half the distance between the electrodes, but there is very little evidence to support this assertion. Bipolar RF is not as penetrating as monopolar RF, so it is not as painful but is often combined with another energy source to increase its efficacy. There are multiple variations of the bipolar RF concept and these are as follows:

1. Fractional or fractionated RF constructed of mini bipolar electrodes (eMatrix, e2, Syneron/Candela, Wayland, MA)
2. Bipolar insulated needle electrodes, which are mechanically inserted into the dermis (ePrime, Syneron/Candela)
3. Bipolar RF combined with other modalities, including diode laser or intense pulsed light (Polaris, Aurora, and Velasmooth, Syneron/Candela)
4. Multiple bipolar electrodes at different distances apart firing sequentially to achieve different depths (EndyMed PRO, EndyMed Medical Ltd, Caesarea, Israel)
5. Bipolar RF with vacuum to control depth of penetration called *functional aspiration controlled electrothermal stimulation* (Aluma, Lumenis Inc, San Jose, CA).

Unipolar

Another form of delivery is unipolar in which there is one electrode, no grounding pad, and a large field of RF emitted in an omnidirectional field around the single electrode. This form is analogous to a radio tower broadcasting signals in all directions. Some devices new to the market are now labeled to be tripolar or multipolar but are variations of the basic 3 forms of monopolar, bipolar, or unipolar. Other energy sources, such as laser or intense pulsed light, can be combined with RF so that a large array of technologies use RF for the ultimate goal of smoothing and tightening of the skin and reduction of fat. Each of these has unique names and marketed advantages.

MONOPOLAR DEVICES
Thermage or ThermaCool

The first device approved for RF skin contraction was the Thermage monopolar RF device, which was cleared by the US Food and Drug Administration (FDA) in 2002 for sale in the United States for general surgical use. In 2004, clearance for periocular wrinkles was obtained. The initial indication that was promoted was treatment of the forehead for eyebrow elevation. Soon after, dermatologists were testing the device for treatment of sagging jowls and skin tightening in other body areas, such as the abdomen and thighs. The US FDA cleared Thermage for body contouring in 2006. Larger handpieces to cover larger areas were also introduced. For ThermaCool, there are 3 components: RF generator, handheld tip with a thin membrane, and a cryogen unit (**Fig. 1**). To deliver cooling, other units use Peltier cooling. Sensors in the thin membrane tip measure temperature and tissue contact. The membrane electrode is designed to disperse energy uniformly across the skin surface in a process termed *capacitive coupling*, which creates a zone of increased temperature at depths of 3 to 6 mm.[6] The depth of heating depends on the size and geometry of the treatment tip.[7] Theoretically, the device heats the dermis from 65C to 75C which is the temperature at which collagen denatures. However, the device protects the epidermis through its cooling apparatus keeping the epidermal temperatures between 35C and 45C. Zelickson and colleagues[3] evaluated the effects of RF (ThermaCool) on 2 samples of human abdominal skin treated with energy ranging from 95 to 181 J. The treatment effect was evaluated using light and electron microscopy of punch biopsies taken immediately and up to 8 weeks after treatment. Immediately after treatment, a mild perivascular and perifollicular infiltrate was observed. At 0, 3, and 8 weeks after treatment, electron microscopy revealed collagen fibrils with greater diameter (shortening of collagen fibers) compared with collagen fibers evaluated before treatment, up to 5 mm deep in the skin.[8] The most recent model, the ThermaCool NXT, has incorporated some of the newer features with several tips; newer handpieces have become available with this new device. These handpieces include tips for the body and eye and a hand piece for cellulite. A new Comfort Plus Technology (Thermage Solta, Hayward, CA) tip is also available, which incorporates massage with RF energy delivery, increasing the speed of the procedure, yet

Table 1
Radio frequency for skin tightening and body contouring

Product/Device	Manufacturer	Frequency	Output Energy	Delivery System	Features
Monopolar Devices					
Exilis	BTL Aesthetics, Prague, CR	3.4 MHz	Up to 120 W/90 W	Contact Cooling	Monopolar energy flow control, safety system, built-in thermometer, no risk of overheating
Thermage	Solta Medical, Hayward, CA	6.78 MHz	400 W	Handpiece with vibration	New hand piece (CPT: Comfortable Pulse Technology) with vibrations to improve patient comfort. Pain nerval interceptors get confused and busy (vibrations, cooling, heating)
Cutera	TruSculpt, Brisbane, CA	1 MHz	N/A	4" hand piece	Hand piece that reads out once optimal temperature is reached of 43–45 degrees C
Ellman	Pelleve, Oceanside, NY	4 MHz Alternating	Levels	4 small hand pieces: 7.5, 10, 15, 20 mm	Several hand pieces for smaller areas. Can use unit as an electro cautery unit also
Biorad	GSD Tech Co, Shenzhen, China	1.15 MHZ	1000 W max	3 tips, one for eyes, face, and body	Continuous cooling; Automatic Resistance Technology; single and continuous mode
Bipolar Devices					
Accent Family	Alma Lasers, Caesarea, Israel	40.68 MHz	Up to 300 W	Multiple devices	Unipolar, bipolar, fractionated
VelaShape II	Syneron/Candela, San Jose, CA	N/A	Infrared- Up to 35 W RF Up to 60 W	Hand piece w/bipolar Radiofrequency, Infrared laser, Suction	Vsmooth (40 mm × 40 mm) and Vcontour (30 mm × 30 mm) treatment areas
eMatrix	Syneron/Candela, San Jose, CA	N/A	Up to 62 mJ/pin	Matrix of electrodes	Disposable tip
Apollo-TriPollar	Pollogen, Tel Aviv, Israel	1 MHz	50 W	3 hand pieces	Large, Medium, Small

Device	Company, Location	Frequency	Power	Configuration	Notes
Reaction	Viora, Jersey City, NJ	0.8, 1.7, 2.45 MHz	Body 50 W Face 20 W	4 modes- 0.8, 1.7, 2.45 + multichannel	SVC (suction, vacuum, cooling)
V-Touch	Viora, Jersey City, NJ	N/A	N/A	3 hand piece-0.8, 1.7, 2.45	SVC (suction, vacuum, cooling)
EndyMEd PRO 3 Deep 3 Pole	EndyMEd Medical, Caesarea, Israel	1 MHZ	65 W	4 hand pieces	3 Deep RF, Handpieces: Skin tightening, body contouring, facial tightening, fractional Skin resurfacing
Venus Concept-8 Circular Poles	Venus Freeze, Toronto, ON	RF: 1 MHz Magnetic pulse: 15 Hz	RF: up to 150-W Magnetic flux: 15 Gauss	Large hand piece 8 poles 5 mm apart, dual mode = bipolar + magnetic field	Multipolar RF and magnetic pulse
TiteFx	Invasix, Yokneam, Israel	1 MHz	60 W	Bi-RF + vacuum	Bipolar w/suction real time epidermal temperature monitor
Aurora SR	Syneron/Candela, San Jose, CA	—	Up to 25 J/cm^3	400–980 nm 580–980 nm 680–980 nm	RF and IPL (Intense pulsed light)
Velasmooth	Syneron/Candela, San Jose, CA	—	700–2000 nm	Handpiece	RF/Infrared light with mechanical manipulation
Aluma	Lumenis Ltd., Yokneam, Israel	40.68 MHz	Up to 300 W	Bipolar and UniLarge handpieces	FACES technology using functional aspiration
Eprime	Syneron/Candela, San Jose, CA	460 ± 5 kHz	84 VRMS	Microneedles	20 degree delivery angle, injected into dermis
eTwo	Syneron/Candela, San Jose, CA	—	62 mJ sublative; 100 J/cm^3 sublime	Matrix of electrodes	RF/Infrared light
Elos Plus	Syneron/Candela, San Jose, CA	1–3 HZ	Variable	8 different applicators	RF/Infrared light
Unipolar Series					
Accent RF	Alma Lasers, Caesarea, Israel	40.68 MHz	Up to 200 W	1 handpiece	Unipolar energy to heat fat, bipolar to deliver energy to dermis
Multipolar Devices					
Vanquish	BTL Aesthetics, Prague, CR	—	—	Non-contact	Operator independent

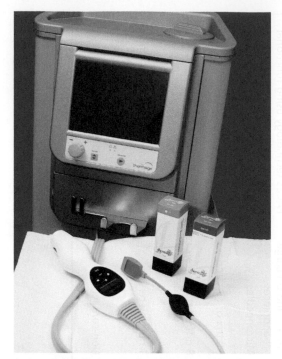

Fig. 1. Thermage unit. The device is equipped to accommodate a large (3 cm) or a small (1 cm) handpiece. Using the larger 3-cm handpiece, it is possible to treat larger areas, like the abdomen.

making it more comfortable by blocking pain using vibration.

Some studies have analyzed the use of RF devices on subcutaneous fat and circumferential reduction in size of treated areas. An interesting study used ThermaCool TC (Solta Medical, Inc, Hayward, CA) device with the Thermage Multiplex Tip to evaluate its effect on abdominal skin laxity and waist circumference.[9] Twelve patients were treated in this study, and the results demonstrated an average decrease in waist circumference of 1.4 cm at the 1-month follow up visit. Another study using a different monopolar RF device was able to demonstrate that adipocyte cell death results from the thermal injury, which was evident starting at 9 days after treatment.[10] Foamy histiocytic and granulomatous infiltrates were observed after cell death around the adipose tissue, but no increase in circulating lipid levels were seen. Jacobson and colleagues[11] treated 24 patients with laxity of the neck, nasolabial folds, marionette lines, and jawline using the ThermaCool system. Each patient received 1 to 3 monthly treatments that consisted of 2 passes on the forehead, 3 on the cheek, and 1 on the neck using 106 to 144 J. Seventeen of the 24 patients showed improvement by 1 month after treatment, but results continued to improve at 3 months after treatment.

Most of the patients described transient burning pain. Patients who underwent multiple treatments and passes had greater results. Alster and Tanzi[12] reported similar findings with the ThermaCool system, with improvement in moderate cheek laxity and nasolabial folds in 30 patients treated with monopolar RF.

Weiss and colleagues[13] published a retrospective chart review to establish the rate and seriousness of side effects and patient satisfaction. More than 600 patients were treated using the ThermaCool device for mild laxity. Patients were treated with multiple passes with fluences of 74 to 130 J/cm^2 using a 1.0-, 1.5-, or 3.0-cm^2 tip. The most common side effects were erythema and edema lasting less than 24 hours. Transient erythema resolved within 5 to 20 minutes, with less than 5% reporting erythema lasting up to 72 hours. The most significant side effects occurred with the original 1-cm^2 tip and included one case of superficial crusting that resolved in 1 week, one case of a slight depression on the cheek that lasted for 3.5 months, 3 cases of subcutaneous erythematous papules, and 3 cases of neck tenderness lasting 1 to 4 weeks. The overall rate of unexpected adverse side effects with the first-generation device was 2.7%; but with subsequent generations and using the multiple-pass lower-energy treatment algorithm, no adverse effects have been seen. Patient satisfaction was high with 90%. Clinical examples of improvement in skin laxity of the face and body are shown in **Figs. 2–4**.

In addition to skin tightening, monopolar RF has also been used to treat active cystic acne to inhibit sebaceous activity and promote dermal contouring. A study including 22 patients with moderate to severe active cystic acne reported improvement with the use of stamped monopolar RF.[14] Patients were treated in 1 to 3 sessions using 65 to 103 J/cm^2. A 75% reduction in the active acne lesion count was seen in 92% of patients, and a 25% to 50% reduction occurred in 9% of patients. Often a decrease in active lesions was accompanied by the improvement of underlying scarring. These results have not been duplicated in other studies.

EXILIS Elite Device

A novel RF dynamic monopolar device, the Exilis, is a device that combines focused monopolar RF delivery with several built-in safety features, including Peltier cooling. The Exilis system delivers the energy through 2 different hand applicators, one designed for the face and one designed for the body (**Fig. 5**). The goal of treatment is to raise the surface temperature to 40°C to 42°C

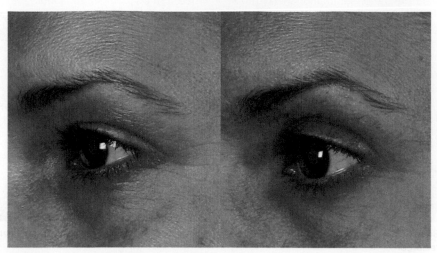

Fig. 2. Before and after Thermage treatment of forehead and eyes showing nice improvement in the laxity of the forehead and eyelid skin.

for 4 to 5 minutes for each region treated. When this temperature is reached, patients feel a comfortably warm sensation. The handpiece is in continuous motion so that the areas of skin with the most laxity can be specifically targeted. This treatment has been termed *dynamic monopolar RF*. Additionally, Peltier cooling can be adjusted up or down to allow targeting of skin or subcutaneous tissue. For example, to drive heating more deeply, the skin is cooled and protected allowing heat to reach into subcutaneous fat. Alternatively, to get the maximum effect on skin laxity, cooling is turned off and heating of the skin occurs very quickly with a minimal effect on subcutaneous fat.

For the body applicator, the temperature is monitored by an on-board infrared temperature sensor, which continuously displays the skin temperature. When the device senses spikes in RF delivery, these spikes are automatically reduced. Constant monitoring of energy flow through tissue (impedance) detects the tip contact with skin. Computerized automatic shutoff of power when the tip contact and/or energy flow is disrupted virtually eliminates the risks of burns, and this is termed the *energy flow control system*. The advantage is that energy flow control allows the use of high power (watts), which then leads to faster treatment times while ensuring the greatest level of safety and comfort.

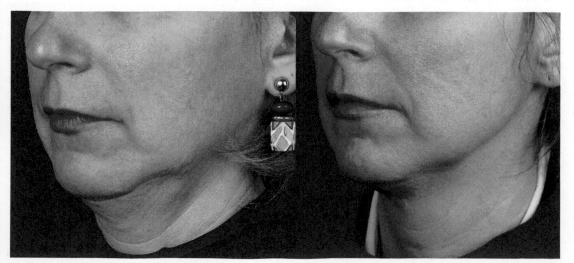

Fig. 3. Before and after Thermage treatment of the lower face and jawline showing nice improvement in skin laxity and increased definition of the jawline.

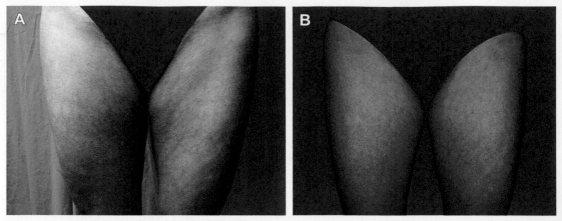

Fig. 4. (*A*). Before treatment. (*B*). After body Thermage treatment of inner thighs. Subtle improvement in skin tone is appreciated.

This device also warns when RF is not being delivered. Experiments have shown that the increased temperature effect is seen as much as 2 cm below the skin with surface cooling (**Fig. 6**). The primary advantage of this system is the ability to target skin laxity or contour deformities. A precise depth of penetration combined with the focused thermal effect caused by advanced controlled cooling allows total-body and full-face applications. A cohort of 30 patients that were treated with the Exilis device on the jowls and neck for rhytid and laxity as well as submental fat pad reduction was followed for 6 months.[15] See clinical example of a facial treatment with Exilis in **Fig. 7**. The age range was 31 to 66 years old. Additionally, 14 of the facial treatment patients were also treated for jiggly fat pads or loose skin on the arms between the shoulder and elbow. The circumference was measured midarm. The

treatment target was fat pad and circumferential reduction and/or tightened skin. Patients were weighed and photographed before and after the study and were instructed to continue with their current lifestyle and not to change their nutrition, caloric intake, or physical activity routines.

The treatment protocols are treatments of 10 minutes for a 20 × 25 cm area, maintaining surface temperatures of 40°C to 42°C, for a total of 4 treatments with each treatment spaced at 7 to 10 days. The skin temperatures at the end of a treatment cycle were typically 40°C, which rapidly decreased at the conclusion of the treatment. The patients were treated lying down comfortably, with the treatment area exposed. Water-based gel (face) or mineral oil (body) was applied to the treatment area before the onset of treatment. The baseline temperature before treatment was typically 32°C.

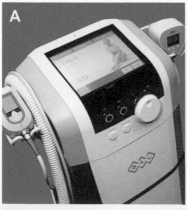
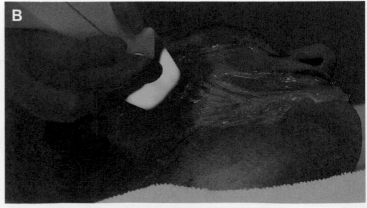

Fig. 5. Exilis unit: Device design for Exilis system (*A*). Unit with 2 handpieces, which includes a body-treatment handpiece with temperature monitoring and a facial-treatment handpiece (*B*). Exilis treatment with the facial handpiece.

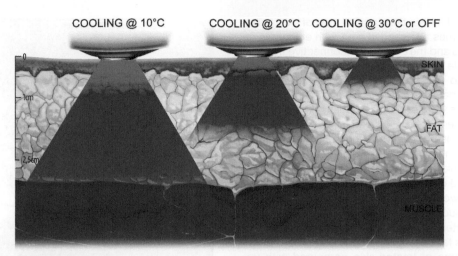

COOLING @ 10°C   COOLING @ 20°C   COOLING @ 30°C or OFF

Fig. 6. Monopolar RF depth can be controlled by cooling; depths of greater than 2 cm can be achieved. (*Courtesy of* BTL, Prague, Czech Republic; with permission.)

The energy and treatment times were adjusted according to the area being treated. For the face, typically 30 W with 100% duty cycle was used. For the body, 50 to 80 W with 100% duty cycle was used. The RF applicator was applied to the skin, maintaining contact with the skin through each 30-second treatment cycle. Circular motions or to-and-fro motions were used to keep the tip moving over the treatment area. The key is not to allow the RF applicator to stop moving but to focus on areas of greatest concern. According to patient feedback, the energy was adjusted up or down, as tolerated, to achieve a sustained surface temperature of 40°C to 42°C with a rapid slope up from the baseline.

In a very recent study using this device, 20 patients had 4 circumferential treatment sessions with the Exilis device for the upper arm.[16] The treatment outcome was not measured by images or circumference but by ultrasound thickness of the fat layer. The measurements were taken at very precise reproducible points on the arm. The investigators reported average posterior fat reduction for the arm of 0.5 cm versus 0.02 for untreated control arms. This finding was a statistically significant measurement of fat reduction by ultrasound fat-layer thickness.

BIPOLAR DEVICES
Aluma

The Aluma is a bipolar RF plus vacuum device that is composed of an RF generator, a handpiece, and a tip with 2 parallel electrodes. When the handpiece with the tip is placed perpendicular to the surface of the skin, the system produces a

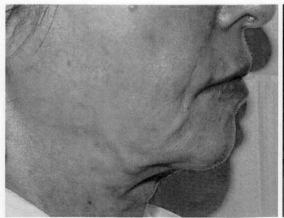

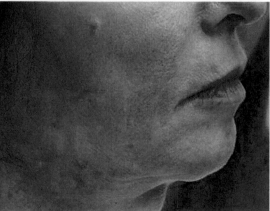

Before Exilis Treatment   **1M after 1 Exilis Treatment**

Fig. 7. Before and after Exilis elite treatment for facial tightening.

vacuum, which suctions a small area of skin.[17] The skin becomes a U-shaped area with epidermis on both sides and the dermis and connective tissue in the middle. The design is to allow the energy emitted to reach the middle and deep dermis. When 46 patients with 8 facial treatments every 1 to 2 weeks were evaluation statistically, significant improvement in facial wrinkles was observed.[18] A low incidence of adverse events, such as burning and crusting, were reported. Another study reported clinical improvement in 30 patients treated with 6 to 8 cycles of the vacuum plus RF system. Patients were treated for multiple clinical conditions, including periocular and glabellar wrinkles, striae distensae, and acne scars. By histology, there was less collagen atrophy and greater interstitial edema of treated skin compared with untreated skin, which showed atrophic dermal collagen with elastotic changes.[19]

eMatrix

Fractional RF is another form of bipolar RF delivery with mini-electrodes. The concept is that RF is omnidirectional so that dots of RF spread out from the point of contact in comparison with laser in which the energy is attenuated in a sharp fashion in interaction with tissue. Fractional RF has been used mainly for skin rejuvenation. Less than 1-mm thermal injuries are formed in a patterned fractional array directly to the reticular dermis. The area directly in contact with and below the array of microneedles or electrodes is selectively heated while the areas between the targeted areas are left intact. A prospective multicenter study was conducted on 35 patients who received 3 treatments on their entire face with a fractional device.[20] Clinical improvement was assessed

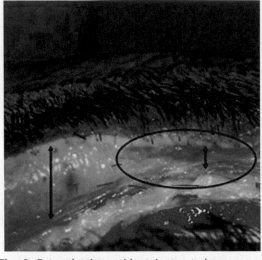

Fig. 9. Fat reduction evident in treated versus untreated area in an animal study using the multipolar noncontact device, Vanquish. The *arrows* show the decrease in width of the fat layer between the treated and nontreated areas of skin.

4 weeks after the last treatment using photographic analysis. Eighty-three percent of patients show improvement in skin brightness, 87% in skin tightness, and 90% in smoothness and wrinkling. Patients undergoing facial treatment had minimal pain and no permanent side effects or significant downtime. The investigators' assessment for improvement in skin texture correlated with the patients' evaluation and was greater than 40% for approximately 50% of the patients. Eighty percent of the patients were satisfied with the results. Higher energy levels and lower coverage rates produced better aesthetic results along with less pain.

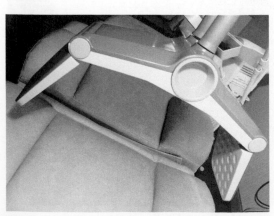

Fig. 8. Vanquish device, a noncontact multipolar device for fat reduction.

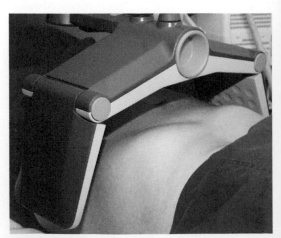

Fig. 10. Patient positioning during a Vanquish treatment.

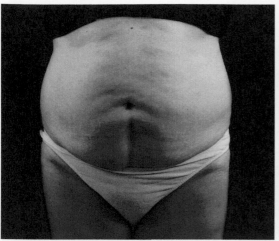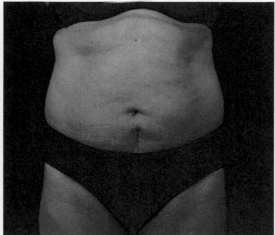

Fig. 11. Clinical improvement in fat reduction before and after a Vanquish treatment series. After 6 treatments of 30 minutes each. (*Courtesy of* Elena Furdeckaj, MD, PEM Clinic of Plastic Surgery, Prague, Czech Republic.)

UNIPOLAR DEVICES
The Accent (Alma Lasers, Inc, Ft Lauderdale, FL)

The Accent RF system is designed for continuous skin contact using 2 handpieces: the unipolar to deliver RF energy to the subcutaneous adipose tissue for volumetric heating and the bipolar to deliver RF energy to the dermis for nonvolumetric heating. It uses both unipolar and bipolar RF and delivers different depths of RF current to the skin, theoretically bipolar for more superficial heating and unipolar for deeper dermal heating. Several clinical trials describe its use in reducing the appearance of cellulite and its effects on tissue tightening.[21–23] In a randomized, blinded, split-design study, 10 individuals (aged 32–57 years) with a clinically observable excess of subcutaneous fat and cellulite (minimum grade 2 out of 4) on the thighs received up to 6 unilateral treatments at 2-week intervals with unipolar RF. All participants responded to a mean of 4.22 treatments with a range of 3 to 6 treatments. Blinded evaluations of photographs using the cellulite grading scale demonstrated 11.25% mean improvement. The treatment was painless; the side effects included minimal to moderate erythema, which resolved within 1 to 3 hours. No crusting, scarring, or dyspigmentation was observed. Clinically visible and quantified improvement, however, did not achieve statistical significance.

MULTIPOLAR NONCONTACT RF DEVICE
Vanquish (BTL Aesthetics, Prague, Czech Republic)

Previously discussed RF devices are operator dependent. This device has been designed for a contactless deep-tissue thermal-energy application (**Fig. 8**). The applicator-generator circuitry is engineered to selectively deliver the energy to the tissue layer with specific impedance. This high-frequency system focuses energy specifically into the adipose tissue, while limiting delivery to the epidermis, dermis, and muscles. Animal studies have shown a 70% fat reduction in the treated abdominal area. Duplex examination demonstrated a reduction of the fat layer from 7.6 to 2.9 mm.[24] Clinical reduction from in the fat layer from the animal study is shown in **Fig. 9**. A series of 4 to 6 treatments are recommended. The device hovers over the abdominal and flank areas (**Fig. 10**). A warm sensation is felt during the 30-minute treatment. It is not painful during or after the procedure. A clinical example of improvement in body fat and contouring is shown in **Fig. 11**.

SUMMARY

Over the past decade, RF has become an important and frequently used technology in cosmetic dermatology. It is most commonly used for tissue heating and tightening as well as body contouring and cellulite reduction. Competitive technologies include vacuum massage, infrared laser technologies, high-frequency focused ultrasound, cavitation frequency ultrasound, and various hybrid energy devices combining some or all of these technologies. RF excites molecules (2–3 million times per second) to create desirable heating effects on collagen and subcutaneous tissues. Many devices use a combination of heat and cooling to noninvasively deliver RF energy to specific depths in tissue, which produces a predictable response, notably collagen remodeling, to achieve desired cosmetic results for wrinkle reduction, tissue tightening, and body contouring. RF currently plays an important role in the authors' practice for the treatment of sagging jowls and mild body contouring. It is a safe technology, which is continually being made safer. Continued research will help to improve the efficacy and increase the knowledge about this rapidly developing technology.

REFERENCES

1. Alster TS, Lupton JR. Nonablative cutaneous remodeling using radiofrequency devices. Clin Dermatol 2007;25:487–91.
2. Weiss R, Weiss M, Beasley K. RF endovenous occlusion. In: Sclerotherapy and vein treatment. 2nd edition. New York (NY): McGraw Hill; 2012. p. 186–95.
3. Zelickson BD, Kist D, Bernstein E, et al. Histological and ultrastructural evaluation of the effects of a radiofrequency-based nonablative dermal remodeling device: a pilot study. Arch Dermatol 2004; 140(2):204–9.
4. Hantash BM, Ubeid AA, Chang H, et al. Bipolar fractional radiofrequency treatment induces neoelastogenesis and neocollagenesis. Lasers Surg Med 2009;41(1):1–9.
5. Bernardy J. Exilis elite effect on subcutaneous tissue. Prague, CR: BTL Aesthetics; 2013. p. 1–7.
6. Bassichis BA, Dayan S, Thomas JR. Use of a nonablative radiofrequency device to rejuvenate the upper one-third of the face. Otolaryngol Head Neck Surg 2004;130(4):397–406.
7. Elsaie ML. Cutaneous remodeling and photorejuvenation using radiofrequency devices. Indian J Dermatol 2009;54(3):201–5.
8. Kist D, Burns AJ, Sanner R, et al. Ultrastructural evaluation of multiple pass low energy versus single pass high energy radio-frequency treatment. Lasers Surg Med 2006;38(2):150–4.
9. Franco W, Kothare A, Ronan SJ, et al. Hyperthermic injury to adipocyte cells by selective heating of subcutaneous fat with a novel radiofrequency device: feasibility studies. Lasers Surg Med 2010;42(5):361–70.
10. Kaplan H, Gat A. Clinical and histopathological results following TriPollar radiofrequency skin treatments. J Cosmet Laser Ther 2009;11(2):78–84.
11. Jacobson LG, Alexiades-Armenakas M, Bernstein L, et al. Treatment of nasolabial folds and jowls with a noninvasive radiofrequency device. Arch Dermatol 2003;139(10):1371–2.
12. Alster TS, Tanzi E. Improvement of neck and cheek laxity with a nonablative radiofrequency device: a lifting experience. Dermatol Surg 2004;30(4 Pt 1):503–7 [discussion: 7].
13. Weiss RA, Weiss MA, Munavalli G, et al. Monopolar radiofrequency facial tightening: a retrospective analysis of efficacy and safety in over 600 treatments. J Drugs Dermatol 2006;5(8):707–12.
14. Ruiz-Esparza J, Gomez JB. Nonablative radiofrequency for active acne vulgaris: the use of deep dermal heat in the treatment of moderate to severe active acne vulgaris (thermotherapy): a report of 22 patients. Dermatol Surg 2003;29(4):333–9 [discussion: 9].
15. Weiss RA. Noninvasive radio frequency for skin tightening and body contouring. Semin Cutan Med Surg 2013;32(1):9–17.
16. Beasley KL, Weiss RA, Weiss MA. Dynamic Monopolar Reduction of Arm Fat by Duplex Ultrasound Imaging and 3D imaging. Lasers Surg Med 2013; 45(S25):20–1.
17. Gold MH. Tissue tightening: a hot topic utilizing deep dermal heating. J Drugs Dermatol 2007; 6(12):1238–42.
18. Gold MH, Goldman MP, Rao J, et al. Treatment of wrinkles and elastosis using vacuum-assisted bipolar radiofrequency heating of the dermis. Dermatol Surg 2007;33(3):300–9.
19. Montesi G, Calvieri S, Balzani A, et al. Bipolar radiofrequency in the treatment of dermatologic imperfections: clinicopathological and immunohistochemical aspects. J Drugs Dermatol 2007;6(9):890–6.
20. Hruza G, Taub AF, Collier SL, et al. Skin rejuvenation and wrinkle reduction using a fractional radiofrequency system. J Drugs Dermatol 2009;8(3):259–65.
21. Alexiades-Armenakas M, Dover JS, Arndt KA. Unipolar radiofrequency treatment to improve the appearance of cellulite. J Cosmet Laser Ther 2008; 10(3):148–53.
22. Emilia del Pino M, Rosado RH, Azuela A, et al. Effect of controlled volumetric tissue heating with radiofrequency on cellulite and the subcutaneous tissue of the buttocks and thighs. J Drugs Dermatol 2006; 5(8):714–22.
23. Alexiades-Armenakas M, Dover JS, Arndt KA. Unipolar versus bipolar radiofrequency treatment of rhytides and laxity using a mobile painless delivery method. Lasers Surg Med 2008;40(7):446–53.
24. Weiss R, Weiss M, Beasley K, et al. Operator independent focused high frequency ISM band for fat reduction: porcine model. Lasers Surg Med 2013; 45:235–9.

New Tattoo Approaches in Dermatology

Stefanie Luebberding, PhD[a],*,
Macrene Alexiades-Armenakas, MD, PhD[a,b]

KEYWORDS

- Tattoo • Tattoo removal • Laser-based tattoo removal • QS laser • Picosecond laser
- Multipass treatments • Dermal scatter reduction

KEY POINTS

- Nonablative and laser-assisted tattoo removal is a frequently performed treatment in today's dermatologic practices.
- Quality-switched ruby, alexandrite, and Nd:YAG laser technologies have been well investigated in numerous randomized and controlled studies and are considered to be the gold-standard for relatively safe and effective tattoo removal.
- Determining the optimal wavelength and treatment modality requires a careful patient evaluation, which must include an assessment of skin type and the tattoo itself.
- Current research in the field of tattoo removal is focused on faster lasers and more effective targeting of tattoo pigment particles in the skin.
- Systematic, randomized, and controlled in vivo studies are required to assess if new innovations are indeed effective and safe.

INTRODUCTION

Body art, such as tattoos, have fascinated mankind for centuries and have already been found in ancient Egyptian, Greek, and Roman cultures. In the past, such body markings served to enhance beauty, provide healing, declare belongings, and were even used to identify criminals and slaves.[1]

The symbolic importance of tattoos has endured through the present day. However, although tattooing in ancient times was a slow and tedious process reserved for a select few, the invention of electric tattooing machines in the 20th century made tattooing available and affordable for the mainstream. Thus, tattoos have become an important part of the modern lifestyle. According to statistics published the Pew Research Center, an American think tank organization, 38% of men and women between the ages of 18 and 29 years

have at least one tattoo. Around 50% of these individuals have 2 to 5 tattoos, whereas 18% indicate that they have 6 or more tattoos.[2] The reasons cited for getting a tattoo include "impulsive decision making", "to be part of a group", "just wanted one", and "for the heck of it", but people also strive for individuality and uniqueness when making such a decision.[3]

Throughout the course of the past 20 years, the prevalence of tattoos has significantly increased. Consequently, the demand for tattoo removal has increased as well. Although surveys suggest that up to 20% of owners may be dissatisfied with their tattoo, 11% consider removal and approximately 6% actually seek tattoo removal.[4] Reasons cited for tattoo removal vary, but patients reported feelings of embarrassment, low self-esteem, problems with clothing, changing of life roles, medical problems, and stigmatization.[1,4,5]

[a] Dermatology and Laser Surgery Center, 955 Park Avenue, New York, NY 10028, USA; [b] Department of Dermatology, Yale University School of Medicine, 333 Cedar Street, LCI 501, PO Box 208059 New Haven, CT 06520, USA
* Corresponding author.
E-mail address: sluebberding@drmacrene.com

Dermatol Clin 32 (2014) 91–96
http://dx.doi.org/10.1016/j.det.2013.09.002

TATTOO REMOVAL

Tattoos are made by inserting indelible ink into the dermis layer of the skin to change the pigment. Although these body marks were once considered to be permanent, the technical and scientific progress in recent years has made it possible to remove tattoos partly or fully by various treatment modalities. Today, tattoo removal is a frequently performed procedure in dermatologic practices.

The methods for tattoo removal can be distinguished into 2 groups, namely ablative and nonablative tattoo removal procedures.

ABLATIVE TATTOO REMOVAL

Historically, several ablative techniques were used to remove tattoos. One of the earliest methods, salabrasion, was introduced by the Greek physician Aetius in 543 AD. Salabrasion is a process incorporating the application of salt and abrasion to rub off the top layers of the skin. Tattoo removal with an abrasive devise was also performed earlier by using dermabrasion, a process by which a wire brush or diamond fraise was used to mechanically abrade the tattooed skin. Another approach used trichloroacetic acid to chemically remove the top layers of the skin up to the dermal layers where the tattoo ink resides.[1,6]

A significant innovation in the area of tattoo removal was the use of lasers in dermatology. In 1965, Leon Goldman first demonstrated the ability of the quality-switched (QS) ruby laser to selectively destroy pigments in the skin.[7] However, because the mechanisms and medical potential for selectively absorbed, high-energy QS lasers were not well understood, the dermatologic use of ruby lasers was abandoned for some time.[8]

In the early 1970s, a variety of continuous lasers were developed for scientific and industrial purposes, including carbon dioxide (far infrared, 10.6-μm wavelength) and argon-ion (Ar-ion; visible spectrum, 488 and 514-nm).[8,9] These laser approaches used water as the targeted chromophore and removed the tattooed skin by ablating the epidermal layers up to the dermis. Ablative carbon dioxide and argon-ion lasers became the treatment of choice for tattoo removal for quite some time.[9]

Although ablative laser treatment modalities for tattoo removal were somewhat successful, they were often accompanied by a wide range of unwanted side effects, including scarring and dyspigmentation. Additionally, the clinical outcome was often unpredictable and results were not satisfying.[10,11] For this reason, the demand for safer and less ablative treatments became evident.

NONABLATIVE TATTOO REMOVAL

The groundbreaking theory of selective photothermolysis, described by Anderson and Parrish[12] in the early 1980s, paved the way for a new generation of laser-based tattoo removal. This theory of selective photothermolysis refers to the precise targeting of chromophores, such as melanin, water, or oxyhemoglobin, using a specific wavelength of light with the intention of absorbing light into the specific target area while leaving surrounding areas relatively untouched.

The method of selective photothermolysis implies that the laser causes targeted heating of exogenous chromophores in the skin, the tattoo pigments, by means of selectively absorbed wavelengths.[13] The high-temperature gradient produced by the laser results in the formation and propagation of acoustic waves that cause mechanical destruction of surrounding structures.[1,14] Therefore, the target chromophore has to be heated very quickly and for no longer than its thermal relaxation time, which is defined as the time required for the target chromophore to lose 50% of its heat.[1,15] Very small structures, such as the tattoo pigment, require rapid heating. In practice this can be accomplished by Q-switching, a technique that produces nanosecond (10^{-9} s) laser pulses by suddenly releasing all of the excited-state energy from the laser medium. Therefore, contemporary technology involves the use of QS lasers[13] that are considered to be the gold-standard treatment option for the removal of unwanted tattoo ink in the skin.[6]

QUALITY-SWITCHED LASERS

The QS ruby laser, introduced by William H. Reid in 1983,[16] was the first commercially available QS laser for tattoo removal, followed by the QS Nd:YAG and QS alexandrite laser. All 3 lasers are still used today in dermatologic practice. However, because the tattooed pigment comes in a wide range of colors, multiple wavelengths of laser light are required to successfully remove tattoos.[1,13]

Studies have shown that dark pigmented tattoos can theoretically be treated by any laser, because black absorbs virtually every wavelength of light.[13] However, Leuenberger and colleagues[17] and others[18-20] found the QS 694-nm ruby and QS 755-nm alexandrite laser to be superior in lightening black-blue tattoos compared with the 1064-nm QS Nd:YAG, but these treatments are frequently associated with transient pigmentary changes, including rare depigmentation. Although the 1064-nm QS Nd:YAG laser is slightly less efficient in the removal of black ink, dyspigmentation and textual changes are much less frequent due to its lower absorption by melanin and keratinocytes in the epidermis; this makes the 1064-nm Nd:YAG laser an excellent choice of therapy for tattoo removal in darker pigmented skin.[21]

The light emitted from the 1064-nm QS Nd:YAG laser may also be frequency-doubled to produce light with a wavelength of 532-nm.[1] Orange, red, and red-brown pigments, in particular, respond well to this wavelength.[18,20,22] The 532-nm option of the QS YAG laser was also found to be superior to the QS 694-nm ruby and the 1064-nm option of the YAG laser in the removal of red colors in professional tattoos.[19,23] The QS 755-nm alexandrite[20] and the QS 694-nm ruby laser[19] were considered the treatment modalities of choice for the removal of green-colored tattoos, whereas purple and violet ink respond best to the QS 694-nm ruby laser.[20]

NEW ADVANCEMENTS IN LASER-ASSISTED TATTOO REMOVAL

Laser-assisted tattoo removal with various QS laser devises still remains the gold-standard therapy in tattoo clearance. However, multiple treatment sessions are required until reaching full or acceptable lightening of the pigmented skin. The number of treatment sessions depends on pigment color, composition, density, depth, age of the tattoo, body location, and the amount of tattoo ink present.[24] On average, 4 to 6 treatment sessions, which are typically spaced 1 to 2 months apart, are required for the complete removal of amateur tattoos, whereas up to 20 sessions are required for professional tattoos.[25,26] Mediocre clinical results as well as prolonged and costly treatment sessions leave more to be desired from both patient and clinician. Therefore, newer unconventional laser-assisted techniques and treatment approaches have been developed to achieve faster and more effective removal of unwanted tattoos.

MULTIPASS TREATMENT

Recently published studies have focused on the possibility to effectively remove tattoos in fewer treatment sessions using a multipass method. In order for this method to be effective, immediate laser-induced cutaneous whitening reactions, likely resulting from thermally induced cavitation bubble formation in the dermis, must subside before delivery of each pass,[24,27] which can be achieved in 1 of 2 ways: either by waiting for spontaneous resolution of whitening reactions, which requires an average of 20 minutes time after each pass (R20 method) or by application of

topical perfluorodecalin (PFD), a highly gas soluble[28] liquid fluorocarbon that resolves the whitening reaction within seconds (R0 method).

In a comparative study, Kossida and colleagues[24] paralleled the efficacy of the conventional single-pass laser tattoo removal, using the 755-nm QS alexandrite laser, to treatment in 4 consecutive passes separated by a 20-minute interval (R20 method). Results demonstrated that the multi-pass R20 method is a safe and far more effective method in lightening tattoos in a single treatment session when compared with conventional single-pass laser treatment. Reddy and colleagues[27] used the QS 694-nm ruby or 1064-nm Nd:YAG laser to compare the conventional single-pass treatment with the R20 and R0 method. Results indicated that the multiple-pass tattoo removal method, using PFD to deliver rapid sequential passes, is as effective as the R20 method, but in a significantly reduced treatment time. Moreover, tattoo clearance of both the R0 and R20 methods are superior to the traditional single-pass laser method with comparable safety potential.

DERMAL SCATTER REDUCTION

Studies have shown that absorption and the natural strong scattering of epidermal and dermal tissue significantly reduce the depth of light penetration and laser energy that may reach the dermal tattoo pigment.[29] This becomes even more evident when treating red, orange, or yellow pigmented tattoos. These inks tend to consist of pigments that need shorter wavelength lasers, such as the 532-nm QS Nd:YAG, whose effectiveness is limited by skin scattering and hemoglobin absorption.[20] However, by temporary reduction of the scattering coefficient of intervening skin layers, increased laser energy and shorter wavelength light may be transmitted more efficiently to the tattoo ink particles in the skin.[30,31]

Therefore, optical-clearing techniques, first introduced by Tuchin and colleagues,[29] may be used to effectively reduce the scattering of dermal tissues by transdermal or intradermal injection of optical-clearing agents (OCAs) with high refractive indices and hyperosmolarity.[32] OCAs such as glycerol, dimethylsulfoxide, and glucose have been shown to significantly reduce dermal scatter in animal models.[32–34] McNichols and colleagues[30] studied the effectiveness of intradermal and transdermal application of glycerol in clearing the skin and compared the outcomes of single-laser treatment sessions for both cleared and uncleared tattoo sites using the QS 755-nm alexandrite and the 532-nm Nd:YAG lasers. Both intradermal and transdermal application of glycerol showed greater tattoo clearance post-laser treatment when compared with the control, particularly for black and light red tattoo pigment. However, intradermal injection was accompanied by a higher risk of necrosis and scarring.

IMIQUIMOD

Histopathologic findings have shown that in acute-phase tattoos, pigments persist partly as free granules in the epidermis and dermis for up to 1 week after ink placement before tattoo maturation has been completed.[35] In this acute phase, pigment response to tattoo removal techniques may be increased.

A recently published study in guinea pigs confirms this assumption and indicates the successful and nonsurgical removal of acute-phase tattoos by topical application of 5% imiquimod cream for 7 days post-treatment.[36] Imiquimod is a topically applied immunomodulator drug that indirectly stimulates both innate immune response as well as cell-mediated acquired immunity.[37] Therefore, imiquimod is believed to interfere with tattoo pigment phagocytosis and prevent tattoo maturation.[36]

A study completed by Taylor and colleagues[38] demonstrated that laser-based tattoo removal was able to recreate the biologic elements of an acute-phase tattoo by inducing phagocytic response and lymphatic transport of ink particles, which were shattered by the laser beam. The efficacy of this method as an adjunct approach for laser-based removal of mature tattoos was confirmed by Ramirez and colleagues[39] in an animal study. The combination of the 755-nm QS alexandrite laser in conjunction with triweekly applications of 5% imiquimod cream showed greater tattoo lightening than laser treatment alone, but involved greater risk for inflammation and fibrosis post-treatment.

Two randomized, double-blind, controlled studies conducted by Ricotti and colleagues[37] and Elsaie and colleagues[40] evaluated the safety and efficacy of topical 5% imiquimod cream used daily in conjunction with laser therapy to remove unwanted tattoos in men. Based on evaluations by both investigators and subjects, Elsaie and colleagues[40] demonstrated more favorable lightening results with the combination therapy. Although Ricotti and colleagues[37] found the results of the QS laser treatment in combination with imiquimod to be slightly superior when compared with control, the research group concluded that topical imiquimod was not effective for laser-assisted tattoo removal due to the significantly higher risk of adverse events.

PICOSECOND LASERS

Most tattoo pigments have a particle size of 30 to 300 nm, corresponding to a thermal relaxation time of less than 10 nanoseconds.[4,41] As it has been previously mentioned, the shorter the pulse length, the more rapid the heating process of the targeted chromophores, and consequently the more effective the removal of the tattooed pigment in the skin. Besides the QS lasers, which offer a pulse duration already in the nanosecond range (10^{-9} s) and newer laser technologies shorten that pulse time to picoseconds (10^{-12} seconds), promising more effective results in tattoo removal.

Fifteen years ago, Ross and colleagues[42] reported that for the same laser energy, tattoo removal becomes more efficient as the laser pulse length is shortened to the picosecond range. In a side-by-side comparison of responses of tattooed pigment to picosecond and nanosecond QS 1064-nm Nd:YAG lasers, Ross and colleagues[42] found that 12 out of 16 black tattoos showed greater lightening with a pulse duration of 35 picoseconds than with a pulse duration of 10 nanoseconds. Similar results were found by Herd and colleagues[25] and Izikson and colleagues[41] who compared the efficacy of the picosecond titanium:sapphire (795-nm, 500 picoseconds) laser and the QS alexandrite (758-nm, 50 nanoseconds) laser in the treatment of tattooed porcine models. Both studies found greater clearance of tattoos treated by picosecond lasers.

The first commercially available picosecond laser, the 755-nm alexandrite laser, was launched in the first quarter of 2013. Recently published studies already confirm the effectiveness of shorter pulse lengths in the treatment of tattoos with safety equivalent to that of QS lasers.[43] Brauer and colleagues[44] described the successful and rapid treatment of 12 tattoos containing blue and/or green pigment with the novel, picosecond, 755-nm alexandrite laser in men. The research group demonstrated at least 75% clearance of blue and green pigment after 1 or 2 treatments, with more than two-thirds of these tattoos more closely approaching 100% clearance.

MICROENCAPSULATED TATTOO INK

Currently, neither the Food and Drug Administration nor any other regulatory authority in the United States regulates the ink and pigment used for tattooing. This implies that there are no legal obligations for manufacturers to disclose pigment ingredients or maintain pharmaceutically pure compositions.[1]

Detailed knowledge with respect to the identity and dye composition of tattoo pigments would be beneficial not only with regard to photo-allergenic, granulomatous, and anaphylactic reactions but will also be useful in improving treatment planning and response prediction to laser therapy.[45] Klitzman[46] designed a permanent but more removable tattoo ink using insoluble and bioresorbable pigments (such as beta-carotene and iron oxide), which are stabilized through microencapsulation in transparent polymethylmethacrylate beads. The microspheres contain discrete pigment that can be targeted by specific laser wavelengths. Laser-based tattoo removal will cause the capsule to break, exposing the pigment, which is then resorbed by the body.[13] Recently presented, unpublished data of Klitzman and colleagues[46] showed significantly increased tattoo removability in hairless rats and guinea pigs. One laser treatment effectively removed 80% of tattoo intensity, whereas only 20% of conventional ink was removed in a single identical laser treatment. Although these results appear promising, the safety and efficacy of microencapsulated tattoo ink in human skin needs to be investigated in further studies as no clinical data have yet been published.

SUMMARY

Nonablative and laser-assisted tattoo removal is a frequently performed treatment in today's dermatologic practices. Thus far, QS ruby, alexandrite, and Nd:YAG laser technologies have been well investigated in numerous randomized and controlled studies and are considered to be the gold-standard for relatively safe and effective tattoo removal. However, each laser has its benefits and to date no generally applicable procedures are yet available; determining the optimal wavelength and treatment modality requires a careful patient evaluation, which must include an assessment of skin type and the tattoo itself.

Current research in the field of tattoo removal is focused on faster lasers and more effective targeting of tattoo pigment particles in the skin. These newer, unconventional modalities include picosecond laser devises, multipass treatments, and microencapsulated tattoo ink. Initial published studies show promising results, which may pave way for safer and more effective laser-based tattoo removal. However, systematic, randomized, and controlled in vivo studies are required to assess if these new innovations are indeed effective and safe.

REFERENCES

1. Kent KM, Graber EM. Laser tattoo removal: a review. Dermatol Surg 2012;38:1–13.
2. Pew Research Center. MILLENNIALS A Portrait of generation next. 2010; 57–58. Available at: http://www.pewsocialtrends.org/files/2010/10/millennials-confident-connected-open-to-change.pdf.
3. Armstrong ML, Roberts AE, Koch JR, et al. Motivation for contemporary tattoo removal: a shift in identity. Arch Dermatol 2008;144:879–84.
4. Bergstrom KG. Tattoo removal: new laser options. J Drugs Dermatol 2013;12:492–3.
5. Klein A, Rittmann I, Hiller KA, et al. An Internet-based survey on characteristics of laser tattoo removal and associated side effects. Lasers Med Sci 2013. [Epub ahead of print].
6. Kirby W, Chen CL, Desai A, et al. Causes and recommendations for unanticipated ink retention following tattoo removal treatment. J Clin Aesthet Dermatol 2013;6:27–31.
7. Goldman L, Wilson RG, Hornby P, et al. Radiation from a Q-switched ruby laser. Effect of reapeted impacts of power output of 10 megawatts on a tattoo of man. J Invest Dermatol 1965;44:69–71.
8. Anderson RR. Dermatologic history of the ruby laser: the long story of short pulses. Arch Dermatol 2003;139:70–4.
9. Reid R, Muller S. Tattoo removal with laser. Med J Aust 1978;1:389.
10. Reid R, Muller S. Tattoo removal by CO laser dermabrasion. Plast Reconstr Surg 1980;65:717–28.
11. Brady SC, Blokmanis A, Jewett L. Tattoo removal with the carbon dioxide laser. Ann Plast Surg 1979;2:482–90.
12. Anderson RR, Parrish JA. Microvasculature can be selectively damaged using dye lasers: a basic theory and experimental evidence in human skin. Lasers Surg Med 1981;1:263–76.
13. Choudhary S, Elsaie ML, Leiva A, et al. Lasers for tattoo removal: a review. Lasers Med Sci 2010;25:619–27.
14. Ho DD, London R, Zimmerman GB, et al. Laser-tattoo removal: a study of the mechanism and the optimal treatment strategy via computer simulations. Lasers Surg Med 2002;30:389–97.
15. Anderson RR, Parrish JA. Selective photothermolysis: precise microsurgery by selective absorption of pulsed radiation. Science 1983;220:524–7.
16. Reid WH, McLeod PJ, Ritchie A, et al. Q-switched Ruby laser treatment of black tattoos. Br J Plast Surg 1983;36:455–9.
17. Leuenberger ML, Mulas MW, Hata TR, et al. Comparison of the Q-switched alexandrite, Nd:YAG, and ruby lasers in treating blue-black tattoos. Dermatol Surg 1999;25:10–4.
18. Kilmer SL, Anderson RR. Clinical use of the Q-switched ruby and the Q-switched Nd:YAG (1064

nm and 532 nm) lasers for treatment of tattoos. J Dermatol Surg Oncol 1993;19:330–8.

19. Levine VJ, Geronemus RG. Tattoo removal with the Q-switched ruby laser and the Q-switched Nd:YAGlaser: a comparative study. Cutis 1995;55: 291–6.

20. Zelickson BD, Mehregan DA, Zarrin AA, et al. Clinical, histologic, and ultrastructural evaluation of tattoos treated with three laser systems. Lasers Surg Med 1994;15:364–72.

21. Jones A, Roddey P, Orengo I, et al. The Q-switched ND: YAG laser effectively treats tattoos in darkly pigmented skin. Dermatol Surg 1996;22:999–1001.

22. Guedes R, Leite L. Removal of orange eyebrow tattoo in a single session with the Q-switched Nd:YAG 532-nm laser. Lasers Med Sci 2010;25:465–6.

23. Ferguson JE, August PJ. Evaluation of the Nd/YAG laser for treatment of amateur and professional tattoos. Br J Dermatol 1996;135:586–91.

24. Kossida T, Rigopoulos D, Katsambas A, et al. Optimal tattoo removal in a single laser session based on the method of repeated exposures. J Am Acad Dermatol 2012;66:271–7.

25. Herd RM, Alora MB, Smoller B, et al. A clinical and histologic prospective controlled comparative study of the picosecond titanium:sapphire (795 nm) laser versus the Q-switched alexandrite (752 nm) laser for removing tattoo pigment. J Am Acad Dermatol 1999;40:603–6.

26. Alster TS. Q-switched alexandrite laser treatment (755 nm) of professional and amateur tattoos. J Am Acad Dermatol 1995;33:69–73.

27. Reddy KK, Brauer JA, Anolik R, et al. Topical perfluorodecalin resolves immediate whitening reactions and allows rapid effective multiple pass treatment of tattoos. Lasers Surg Med 2013;45:76–80.

28. Mackanos MA, Jansen ED, Shaw BL, et al. Delivery of midinfrared (6 to 7-microm) laser radiation in a liquid environment using infrared-transmitting optical fibers. J Biomed Opt 2003;8:583–93.

29. Tuchin VV, Maksimova IL, Zimnyakov DA, et al. Light propagation in tissues with controlled optical properties. J Biomed Opt 1997;2:401–17.

30. McNichols RJ, Fox MA, Gowda A, et al. Temporary dermal scatter reduction: quantitative assessment and implications for improved laser tattoo removal. Lasers Surg Med 2005;36:289–96.

31. Fox MA, Diven DG, Sra K, et al. Dermal scatter reduction in human skin: a method using controlled application of glycerol. Lasers Surg Med 2009;41:251–5.

32. Wen X, Mao Z, Han Z, et al. In vivo skin optical clearing by glycerol solutions: mechanism. J Biophotonics 2010;3:44–52.

33. Yoon J, Son T, Jung B. Quantitative analysis method to evaluate optical clearing effect of skin using a hyperosmotic chemical agent. Conf Proc IEEE Eng Med Biol Soc 2007;2007:3347–9.

34. Vargas G, Chan KF, Thomsen SL, et al. Use of osmotically active agents to alter optical properties of tissue: effects on the detected fluorescence signal measured through skin. Lasers Surg Med 2001;29:213–20.

35. Hurwitz JJ, Brownstein S, Mishkin SK. Histopathological findings in blepharopigmentation (eyelid tattoo). Can J Ophthalmol 1988;23:267–9.

36. Solis RR, Diven DG, Colome-Grimmer MI, et al. Experimental nonsurgical tattoo removal in a guinea pig model with topical imiquimod and tretinoin. Dermatol Surg 2002;28:83–6.

37. Ricotti CA, Colaco SM, Shamma HN, et al. Laser-assisted tattoo removal with topical 5% imiquimod cream. Dermatol Surg 2007;33:1082–91.

38. Taylor CR, Anderson RR, Gange RW, et al. Light and electron microscopic analysis of tattoos treated by Q-switched ruby laser. J Invest Dermatol 1991;97: 131–6.

39. Ramirez M, Magee N, Diven D, et al. Topical imiquimod as an adjuvant to laser removal of mature tattoos in an animal model. Dermatol Surg 2007;33: 319–25.

40. Elsaie ML, Nouri K, Vejjabhinanta V, et al. Topical imiquimod in conjunction with Nd:YAG laser for tattoo removal. Lasers Med Sci 2009;24:871–5.

41. Izikson L, Farinelli W, Sakamoto F, et al. Safety and effectiveness of black tattoo clearance in a pig model after a single treatment with a novel 758 nm 500 picosecond laser: a pilot study. Lasers Surg Med 2010;42:640–6.

42. Ross V, Naseef G, Lin G, et al. Comparison of responses of tattoos to picosecond and nanosecond Q-switched neodymium: YAG lasers. Arch Dermatol 1998;134:167–71.

43. Saedi N, Metelitsa A, Petrell K, et al. Treatment of tattoos with a picosecond alexandrite laser: a prospective trial. Arch Dermatol 2012;148:1360–3.

44. Brauer JA, Reddy KK, Anolik R, et al. Successful and rapid treatment of blue and green tattoo pigment with a novel picosecond laser. Arch Dermatol 2012;148:820–3.

45. Timko AL, Miller CH, Johnson FB, et al. In vitro quantitative chemical analysis of tattoo pigments. Arch Dermatol 2001;137:143–7.

46. Klitzman B. Development of permanent but removable tattoos. First international conference on tattoo safety. BfR-Symposium. Berlin, June 7, 2013.

Robotic Hair Restoration

Paul T. Rose, MD, JD*, Bernard Nusbaum, MD

KEYWORDS

- Follicular unit extraction • Follicular isolation technique • Robotic hair transplantation
- Follicular units • Transection • Strip harvesting

KEY POINTS

- The robotic system of hair restoration is an important addition to the techniques used for hair restoration surgery.
- Robotic hair restoration is based on the follicular unit extraction/follicular isolation technique (FUE/FIT) harvesting process and provides the means to obtain such grafts in a reliable and efficient manner while maintaining low transection rates.
- The advantages and disadvantages associated with the robotic device are similar to those of manual or mechanized FUE/FIT harvesting.
- Using the robotic system a physician can more easily add hair replacement to his or her practice and not have to markedly increase staffing.

INTRODUCTION

The use of robotic mechanisms that assist in surgery have been available for more than two decades. The most prominent system is the Da Vinci system (Intuitive, Sunnyvale, CA) whereby a physician directs the movement of the robotic apparatus in various surgical procedures.

An advantage of a robotic system is that it can perform repetitive maneuvers with great precision. This ability to perform repetitive movement lends itself particularly well to the performance of hair restoration procedures when follicular unit extraction/follicular isolation technique (FUE/FIT) is used. The robot assumes some of the tasks that would require several assistants if a strip harvesting procedure is undertaken. The system also requires less time to be proficient with FUE/FIT compared with learning to do manual FUE/FIT surgery.

The ARTAS system (Restoration Robotics, Sunnyvale, CA) is a robotic device developed specifically for the FUE/FIT procedure. It is cleared by the Food and Drug Administration (FDA) and approved for use only in men for the purpose of hair transplantation.

FUE/FIT is a form of follicular unit grafting[1] and is a technique for removing hair grafts based on obtaining intact follicular units[2] or intact parts of a follicular unit from the donor area of a patient's scalp and then implanting the grafts into appropriate recipient sites (**Figs. 1** and **2**). The technique is essentially the old fashioned punch-graft procedure[3] but performed with small punches, usually 0.7 to 1.2 mm in size. Whereas the 4- or 5-mm punches used in the older punch technique harvested multiple follicular units, which may or may not have been totally intact, the FUE/FIT process is designed to remove single follicular units or intact parts of a follicular unit.[4–6]

The primary attraction for patients who seek FUE/FIT is that it is considered to be a less invasive or minimally invasive procedure compared with strip harvesting and most importantly, a linear scar is avoided. The patient may be able to wear his hair shorter than if a strip harvest was performed but there is a limitation to this, because

Disclosures: Dr Rose has been a consultant to Restoration Robotics; Dr Rose owns stock in Restoration Robotics; Drs Rose and Nusbaum have an ARTAS system in their office.
Hair Transplant Institute Miami, 4425 Ponce de Leon Boulevard, Suite 230, Coral Gables, FL 33146, USA
* Corresponding author.
E-mail address: paultrose@yahoo.com

Dermatol Clin 32 (2014) 97–107
http://dx.doi.org/10.1016/j.det.2013.09.008

derm.theclinics.com

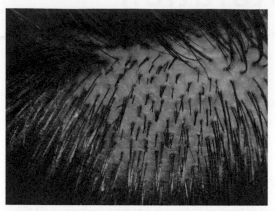

Fig. 1. Normal appearance of hairs in the scalp. It is important to notice that the hairs generally occur in groupings, referred to as "follicular units."

the wounds from FUE can be visible if the head is closely shaved. The appearance of the scar from strip harvesting depends on multiple factors, such as donor density, strip width, tension on closure, scalp laxity, surgical technique, and the patient's healing characteristics.

Some advocates of FUE/FIT believe that the recovery time is shorter and patients can assume strenuous activities sooner.[7] They also suggest that the procedure is less painful than with strip harvesting. The wounds from FUE do tend to appear closed in 4 to 5 days, whereas a strip harvest patient has sutures or staples in place for 7 to 14 days.

The FUE/FIT procedure is considered well suited for a young patient who is uncertain as to whether he will ever want to shave his scalp or proceed with additional hair transplants. If he were to have a strip harvest, concealing the resultant scar

could be a possible concern. Thus, the FUE technique gives the patient more flexibility in the future as to whether to have more procedures. FUE is also very helpful when the scalp is tight in the donor area after strip harvesting and therefore the number of grafts that can be obtained with further strip procedures is limited. FUE/FIT can also be very useful in obtaining grafts for insertion into existing linear strip harvest scars. FUE/FIT can also be used to harvest body hairs.[8]

In regard to postoperative pain, the authors have found that with strip harvesting pain is well controlled with medication, such as oxycodone. Furthermore, with the use of liposomal-encapsulated bupivicaine (Exparel; Pacira Pharmaceuticals, Parsippany, NJ) postoperative pain is less commonly an issue with strip harvesting. The liposomal-encapsulated bupivicaine lasts up to 72 hours.

For the physician, an advantage to performing FUE is that fewer personnel are required compared with strip harvesting. This is because large strip harvest cases require several assistants to dissect the follicular unit grafts from the harvested donor strip tissue. With FUE, the procedure can be done with only one or two additional assistants whose role is to simply clean the grafts and sort them into follicular unit groups containing one, two, or three or more hairs.

The manual technique involves using a biopsy punch of some type and manually harvesting the follicular unit grafts. Many physicians use a sharp punch, whereas some use a combination of a sharp punch to enter the epidermis and then a dull punch to go into the dermis and fat.[6,9] Some physicians use a motorized drill with a punch attachment for this type of harvesting.[10] There are several variations of a motorized drill on the market (Fig. 3). The use of a motorized drill

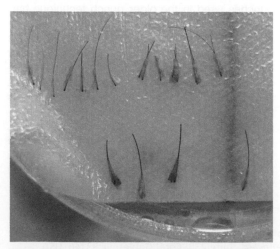

Fig. 2. Follicular unit grafts are depicted. Typically the grafts contain one hair, two hairs, or three hairs. On occasion follicular units with greater numbers of hairs in the unit occur.

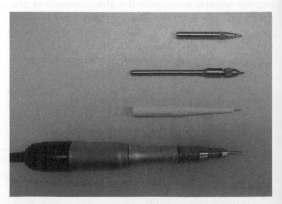

Fig. 3. Different types of punches used to harvest FUE/FIT grafts. A motorized drill with a punch is also shown.

can help skilled physicians harvest quickly and maintain low transections rates, with some physicians attaining harvest rates in excess of 400 grafts per hour with transection rates below 10%. It can be difficult, however, for some clinicians to develop the necessary skill set to attain low transection rates and adequate speed to perform the procedure efficiently. Additionally, FUE can be a tedious and tiring procedure for physician and patient.

At times transection rates can be quite high. In one FDA study the transection rate of manual FUE was noted to be about 26%, whereas the robotic procedure was rated to be 8%.[7,11] The authors have found lower transection rates with their approach to FUE/FIT and believe that physicians can develop the skill to accomplish lower transection rates with the manual process than that reported by the FDA. In the authors' own experience the transection rate for the robot can exceed 8%.

As a side note, it is important to make sure that the definition of transection rate is agreed on by all surgeons performing FUE. The author defines transection as a graft where any of the target hairs are severed. If the surgeon attempts to obtain a three-hair graft and harvests only two of the hairs while the third hair is damaged, then a transection has occurred. Some define a transection as a graft where none of the hairs were obtained.

THE ROBOTIC SYSTEM

The robotic system is FDA approved for male patients with brown or black hair. It consists of a proprietary imaging technology, computer interface terminal, multiple video cameras, video display, the robotic arm device, a suction system to lift up the harvested grafts, and an ergonomic chair that positions the patient in the proper orientation for the robot. The chair is adjustable for height, rotation, and head position (**Fig. 4**).

The robot scans and digitizes the visual characteristics of the donor area and characterizes each follicular unit. Based on a mathematical algorithm that can be adjusted to some extent, the machine randomly harvests follicular units.[12–14] Spacing is such that the harvested grafts are adequately spaced apart so as to decrease the chance that the graft sites would be visible if the patient wears his hair quite short. The computer program also calculates follicular unit density and hair angulation.

The robotic arm has a dual-bore needle apparatus that includes a sharp needle tip to enter the skin and a surrounding coring blunt needle that then goes deeper into the tissue to limit the chance

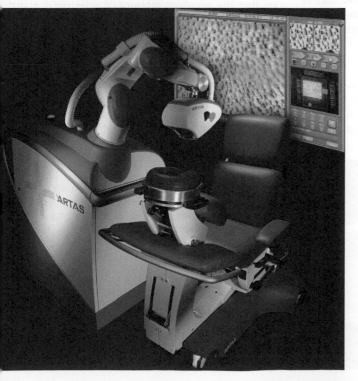

Fig. 4. The Restoration Robotics ARTAS system includes the robotic arm, ergonomic chair, and video monitors. (*Courtesy of* Restoration Robotics, Inc, San Jose, CA; with permission.)

of transection of hairs and allow for easier removal of the selected follicular units. The sharp needle has graduated markings to allow the physician to assess the depth of penetration.

The system is designed for use by a physician in conjunction with an assistant working at a computer terminal. Together the physician and assistant can continually make adjustments as needed to facilitate harvesting.

The robotic system has pressure sensors that assess forces generated to penetrate tissue. The system ceases operation and requires a resetting of the parameters if the threshold of force needed to penetrate the tissue is exceeded. The device has several other safety features. The safety system of the robot prohibits the robotic arm from touching other parts of the robotic arm that might hinder advancement of the needle apparatus or cause damage to the robotic arm. The robot is designed to prevent any possible injury to the patient by restricting the movement of the arm if necessary. It is noted that more than 350 patients were treated in the clinical trials and there were no safety-related issues.[15] The physician and assistant have emergency stop buttons to cease operation of the machine. The emergency stop button is located on the "pendant" handpiece that the physician uses to control the various functional parameters of the device (Fig. 5).

Patient movements are monitored by the robotic system allowing the machine to move to some extent with the patient. If movement is excessive the robot indicates that it cannot adequately recognize the follicular units and ceases harvesting.

THE ROBOTIC PROCEDURE
Medical and Surgical History

As with other surgical procedures the patient's medical and surgical history are obtained before the procedure. A diagnosis of male-pattern hair loss is confirmed by appropriate examination. In some cases the diagnosis of a hair loss condition apart from male-pattern hair loss may also be suitable for hair transplantation. Depending on physician preference, laboratory work, such as complete blood count, complete metabolic profile, prothrombin time and partial thromboplastin time, and hepatitis and HIV status, may be obtained before surgery.

Preoperative Photographs and Marking

At the time of the surgery, photographs are taken of the patient's scalp from the front, sides, back, and top of the head. Appropriate informed consent is provided.

The recipient area is designed and marked and then the area to be harvested is marked out and shaved to a length of approximately 2 mm. Photographs are once again taken to demonstrate the recipient area design and the marked donor area.

In most patients the proposed donor area conforms to the safe area of hairs that are expected to survive throughout the patient's life.[16] In some instances the physician may decide to harvest outside of the recognized safe area if he or she believes that the patient's hair loss will be limited and allow removal of grafts from beyond the safe zone.

The authors often divide the donor area into sections. Usually four sections are marked out, two central portions and two lateral portions. The area to be harvested is anesthetized in sections so that the smallest amount of anesthetic agent is used at any one time throughout the course of the surgery. The authors use 1% lidocaine with epinephrine 1:100,000 for this purpose.

Anesthetic

The patient is typically provided some form of sedation, such as diazepam or similar medication. Pain medication may also be given. Some

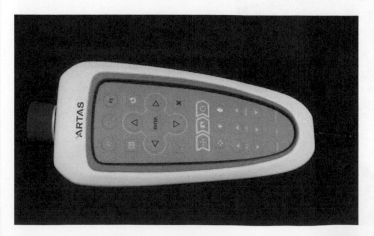

Fig. 5. The "pendant" that is held by the physician provides an ability to adjust the various harvesting parameters of the robotic device. There is an emergency stop button should the physician need to stop the machine while in motion.

physicians elect to give preoperative antibiotics routinely, whereas some give antibiotics depending on the patient's health status. Some physicians use intravenous sedation, which allows for easier maneuverability of the patient and limits ill-timed patient movements that slow down the use of the robotic device.

Robotic Technique

- After the patient is positioned in the chair, in a semiprone orientation, the surgeon applies a tensioner to the initial area selected to be harvested. The tensioner measures approximately 10 to 11 cm^2 and it is crucial that the skin be stretched before application of the tensioner and that the tensioner be placed securely on the desired area (**Fig. 6**).
- To increase the rigidity of the tissue in the area, fluid, such as saline or saline with epinephrine 1:100,000, is injected into the dermis to provide a firmer surface so that the robot can incise into the skin more easily.
- The physician works with an assistant stationed at a computer terminal. The robot is then directed to identify borders of the tensioner (**Fig. 7**). The tensioner has fiducial markings that allow the robot to track patient movement and ensure proper alignment for the robot to recognize the area and the grafts in the enclosed space. With the tensioner in place the robot then scans the image of the enclosed donor area. The robotic cameras then send the image to the computer to recognize the follicular units, angle of hairs, and the follicular unit density within the tensioner area (**Fig. 8**).
- After the follicular units are identified the robot can then begin to select units for harvesting. The robot determines the angle of the hair

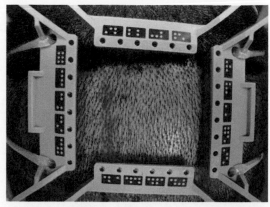

Fig. 7. The tensioner is positioned onto the skin for donor harvesting. The fiducial markings are seen along the periphery of the tensioner. These marking allow for orientation of the robot by the imaging system.

follicles and a suitable angle for the robotic needle to approach the follicular unit. The surgeon can control the machine by a "pendant" that has various buttons controlling the harvesting parameters (see **Fig. 5**). The person operating the computer terminal, which can be the physician or an assistant, also has the ability to control some aspects of the harvesting process. In the course of harvesting the physician has the ability to select or skip units chosen by the robot.

- The robotic arm has at its end a sharp 1-mm needle that initially penetrates or "scores" the skin, just entering the epidermis. This portion of the needle has clearly visible gradation markings on the monitor to allow the physician to control the depth of penetration. A second blunt punch then enters the skin to a greater depth to core out the graft. The depth of the needle penetration and the depth of the coring blunt punch can be adjusted as needed by the physician. Additionally, the speed of the drill tip can be adjusted. The vacuum assist helps to raise the grafts up facilitating harvesting and also allows visualization of the harvested grafts below their epidermal surface to adjust parameters and optimize graft quality.
- After several grafts have been incised, the physician assesses from the video screen the quality of the graft harvesting (**Fig. 9**). Several grafts can also be examined by collecting them from the tensioner enclosed area. If the physician is satisfied with the grafts the robot can be placed on automatic mode and the machine will harvest at speeds generally ranging from 300 to 500 grafts per hour.

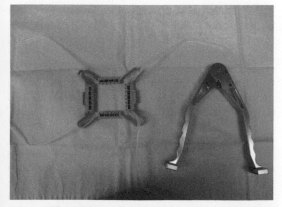

Fig. 6. The tensioner and the tool used to place the tensioner onto the donor skin.

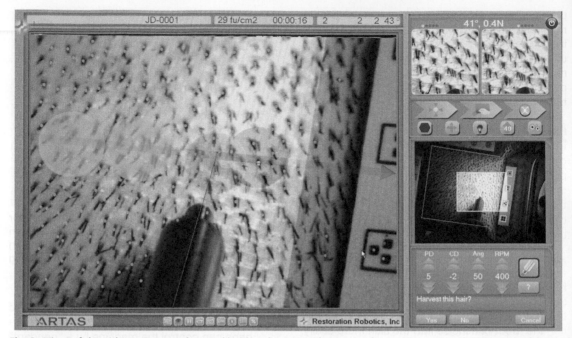

Fig. 8. View of the video screen as observed by the physician. The screen shows parameters that are considered to harvest the tissue. CD, coring depth of the outer blunt needle; PD, punch depth of the needle. The speed of rotation can be adjusted (RPM) and the angle of attack can also be observed on the video screen. (*Courtesy of* Restoration Robotics, Inc, San Jose, CA; with permission.)

Graft harvest speeds in excess of these numbers are reported.

- After the initial tensioner area is harvested the tensioner is removed and the grafts are collected, examined, and trimmed under a microscope if necessary. The tensioner is then moved to an adjacent area and the same process discussed previously is repeated. Logistically, it may be helpful to harvest several grids and collect the grafts while another grid is operated on. At times the suction component may not be able to elevate the incised grafts. Such grafts are often tethered to underlying tissue and it may be necessary to free up the graft. Using a 19-gauge needle can be helpful in releasing the graft.

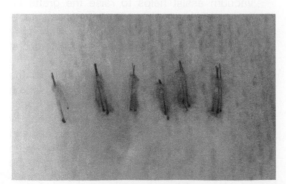

Fig. 9. Typical grafts harvested by the robotic device.

An average Norwood type V or VI patient is able to have 1500 to 2000 grafts harvested in a single session. Some physicians have reported harvesting in excess of 3000 grafts from some patients. In such instances the patient may have a particularly high follicular unit density, large head, and therefore an extended surface area of harvesting available. It may be that the surgeon has decided to exceed the safe donor zone and/or grafts are cut down to smaller sizes.

It is noted that graft harvest speed is not directly correlated to the time it takes to complete the procedure. Graft harvest speeds apply only to the rate the robot is incising grafts at the time it is in the automatic mode. Time is added by having to manually collect the grafts, reposition the tensioner, make recipient sites, and place grafts. Therefore, if 1500 grafts could actually be harvested in 3 hours there would still be several additional hours needed to place all the grafts in the recipient site. A 1500-graft case might take 5 to 6 hours to complete.

Recipient Site

After the grafts are collected they are placed into recipients sites. This step is performed in the identical fashion as when follicular unit transplantation grafts are obtained from strip harvesting. The recipient sites are made for one-, two-, three-, and four-hair follicular units. Many physicians make recipient sites with custom-cut blades ranging from 0.7 to 1.5 mm in size. Others use premade blades or use needles, such as a 19-gauge, to make recipient sites. The same aesthetic considerations are followed as with any other hair restoration procedure.

Some physicians elect to make some or all of the recipient sites the day before the procedure to shorten the operative time on the subsequent operative day. This means that the surgeon has predetermined to a large extent the number of one-, two-, and three-hair grafts and what size the recipient sites will be before knowing for certain what the sizes of the harvested follicular units are at the actual time of surgery.

Postoperative

Postoperatively patients apply antibiotic ointment and alternate with a water-soluble lubricating jelly to the donor area. After 1 week we suggest the use of a product such as Mederma (Merz Pharmaceutical, Greensboro, NC).

Advantages

The use of a robotic device to perform FUE can be advantageous for various reasons. The procedure done manually requires significant skill that can take a substantial time to learn because the surgeon must account for hair direction, exit angle, density of skin, and selection of grafts. The process itself can be physically taxing for the physician. These issues are resolved with the use of the robot because it excels at such repetitive actions. The robot obviously does not experience fatigue and it has sufficient accuracy to ensure acceptable transection rates. The learning curve for proper use of the robotic device is significantly shorter than that for learning manual FUE/FIT.

For a physician entering the field of hair restoration an important advantage of the robotic procedure is that fewer personnel are needed compared with a strip harvest.[11] An assistant is used to help manipulate the robot by a computer terminal. At the same time the physician directs the device and is able to control the various parameters for harvesting.[14] The grafts recovered have a small amount of tissue on them so that further trimming is minimal, if needed at all. The placement of the grafts can be done by the surgeon and the assistant or in most instances two assistants place the harvested grafts.

From a patient point of view the robotic device advantages are akin to FUE/FIT whether manual or robotic. It is a procedure that is ideal for a patient who is averse to an incision and the idea of

a linear scar. In a young patient who is uncertain as to whether he may want to have multiple hair transplant procedures or simply shave the scalp in the future, the robotic technique provides an ability to be more flexible in decision making. The patient can have a procedure and perhaps later decide not to have any more procedures, yet still be able to wear his hair quite short without evidence of a surgical procedure in the donor area. The patient would probably be reluctant to shave his head because the remnants of the punch wounds might be evident as hypopigmented dots.

The wounds with FUE seem to heal more quickly compared with strip harvesting where the donor site is sutured. There may be less postoperative pain in the first 24 hours but this may be a moot issue with the author's use of liposomal marcaine in strip surgery.

With strip harvesting there can be a period of tightness and paresthesia in the donor area, whereas a sense of tightness generally does not occur with the robotic procedure or FUE/FIT. In general, there may be a lower incidence of postoperative parasthesias but these seem to be of little consequence in strip harvesting because the parasthesias are infrequent and resolve quickly. Because no sutures are used with robotic harvesting or FUE/FIT there is no suture removal discomfort and one less visit to the clinic.

For the patient with a naturally occurring very tight scalp or tightness because of previous surgery, FUE/FIT is often the preferred way to harvest grafts and ensure avoiding a wide scar yet still harvest a significant number of grafts. Similarly, some patients have natural thinning in the supraauricular area. That could allow a linear scar to be conspicuous. The FUE/FIT technique may allow harvesting without the possible appearance of linear scarring.

Disadvantages

As with any procedure there are advantages and disadvantages. The disadvantages of the robotic procedure are few but the physician needs to be aware of them. The robotic system relies on the machinery being able to adjust to patient movement and the ability to harvest along a curved surface, the skull. If the patient is moving to a great extent the robotic system will have difficulty properly aligning and a considerable time can be expended before the harvesting can occur. The sweet spot for manual FUE is generally believed to be the center occipital area and this is also true for robotic harvesting. As the harvesting moves to the lateral areas, particularly supraauricular areas, the angle of hair growth can be difficult for the robot to align with and transection rates tend to be somewhat higher. Areas of varying hair direction can be a problem for the robot and working in the softer tissue of the nape yields reduced numbers of viable grafts, as is also true with manual FUE.

With continued harvesting (often multiple sessions) one notices with FUE and probably with robotic surgery that it becomes increasingly arduous to harvest large amounts of hair and higher transection rates may result from hair angle changes that result from adjacent scar tissue.

With manual FUE the surgeon can pick out particular grafts or particular types of grafts, such as two- or three-hair follicular units. This is much more difficult to do with the robot; however, recent changes to the software may allow this to be accomplished.

As with manual FUE/FIT, it is more difficult to harvest curly and particularly kinky hair as seen in blacks. In such situations or in situations where transection rates are unacceptable the surgeon may need to abandon the procedure and possibly perform strip harvesting if the patient has so consented.

Because the robot is a complex and sophisticated device with a computer interface there is a potential for mechanical, software, or hardware breakdown. If this should occur the surgeon needs to stop the procedure and have the patient return when the problem is fixed or have the patient consider manual FUE or even a strip procedure.

Because studies for the robotic system were done on males the FDA has approved its use to only male patients. Also, because the robotic system relies on the contrast between hair and the skin to identify hair clusters the system is only approved for use in patients with brown or black hair. If the patient has white or very blond hair this issue can be overcome by dyeing the patient's hair.

Although FUE/FIT is often advertised as a no scar or minimal scar procedure the mathematics prove otherwise.[17,18] The wounds created by FUE whether robotic or from manual FUE produce round scars where little or no hair grows. These spots are often hypopigmented and larger than the punch diameter used. If the patient wears his hair quite short or shaved, the scalp has an appearance of having been struck by buckshot (**Fig. 10**).

Although a 1-mm punch may be used for harvesting the resultant scar is often greater than 1 mm and may approach 2 mm or more. If one takes 1000 grafts and calculates the area of scar even with 1-mm circles the area is $1000 \times pi \times$ radius squared. This equals 7.85 cm². For the same number of grafts a linear scar in a patient

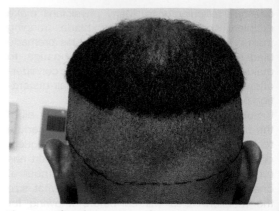

Fig. 10. After harvesting of FUE/FIT graft whether manually or with a drill or robotic device the donor wound scars may hypopigment leaving a buckshot appearance to the donor area.

with 80 follicular units per square centimeter density, scar length of 12.5 cm, and a scar width of 2 mm, the total area would be 2.5 cm. Thus, the total area of scar created with FUE is generally greater than with strip harvesting given the same amount of grafts harvested.

As with other forms of FUE, if there is continued harvesting in successive sessions the donor area becomes thin and less dense. There can be a "step off" from the harvested donor safe area to the zone above that has not been harvested and is at least temporarily denser. For this reason it may be wise to perform low-density harvesting into the more superior areas to blend the densities of the safe donor area with the more superior hair.

When multiple sessions or excessive harvesting takes place, the donor area can have a moth-eaten appearance. Again, this is not a problem associated with the robotic device but rather the FUE approach, because nothing is being put back in place of the hairs taken out of the donor area. The author has used suction applied to the wounds to further improve healing of FUE/FIT wounds and decrease the size of the scars.

An issue inherent to FUE is that fewer grafts can generally be harvested in a single session compared with strip harvesting. This is because, to allow for adequate spacing between extraction sites, the surgeon can only remove approximately 12% to 20% of the grafts available in the first harvest session without the human eye detecting the pattern of wounds if the hair is cut very short.[17] With subsequent sessions the percentage that can be harvested decreases further. There have been reports from several doctors using the robotic system of cases in excess of 3000 grafts in one session. It seems that the surgeon is going beyond the traditional safe donor zone and may be cutting down grafts to smaller sizes.

The author has observed that the robotic system does not seem to work well in patients with previous strip harvesting. The area around the scar is often significantly less dense and the area of fibrosis makes it difficult for the robot to penetrate the skin. Also, the hair direction may be altered in the area adjacent to the scar and so transection rates may increase.

When large numbers of grafts are needed, the robotic surgery can be tiring for the patient. Some patients feel a sense of claustrophobia in the chair. There are patients who simply move too much for harvesting to proceed at a reasonable rate and acquire high-quality grafts. These patients tend to be very anxious at the outset and such patients might be best suited for having the procedure performed with intravenous sedation in an appropriate facility.

ADVERSE REACTIONS AND COMPLICATIONS

The complications associated with robotic surgery are essentially the same as with any FUE process.[18]

Buried Grafts

At times the use of a small-diameter punch inadvertently pushes the incised tissue further into the skin. The result is a graft that is buried in the adipose tissue. Oftentimes these grafts tend to be pushed off to the side adjacent to the incision. The surgeon can attempt to find the graft by probing the area with a mosquito hemostat or forceps. Making an incision with a #11 blade into the space created from attempting to remove the graft and pushing down on the surrounding tissue may force the graft upward and outward, allowing recovery of the graft. Sometimes injecting saline into the area may push the graft out. If one is unable to retrieve the graft, it is left alone. If the graft remains buried there may be a subsequent foreign body reaction or possibly a cyst may form and may need drainage or excision.

Transection

Transection results in damaged hair follicles and in some instances entire follicular unit grafts that are not usable. Some physicians argue that transection may not be important but could be beneficial because some hair might regrow at the FUE wound site. This would serve to camouflage to some extent the harvesting that has been performed. The surgeon should be aware of the degree of transection throughout the procedure and

make adjustments of the various parameters of the robotic system to remedy the problem should it occur.

Although most physicians would agree that transection should be kept to a minimum, the question of what is an acceptable rate is crucial. Many who perform manual FUE believe that transection rates less than 10% are reasonable.

Thinning of the Donor Area Hair

As a result of FUE harvesting, the wounds result in areas in which no hairs grow. If the patient elects to wear his hair very short the resultant scars may be evident as an appearance of multiple dots with no hair, reminiscent of buckshot wounds. In some areas where the grafts have been harvested in close proximity in one or multiple sessions there can be a visible thinning of the hair in the donor area and a step off of hair density from the higher density above the harvest zone. There may also be an impression of a moth-eaten appearance to the scalp in areas where concentrated harvesting has occurred.

Hypopigmentation and Hyperpigmentation

The scars that occur with FUE whether by robotic device or manual harvesting are usually hypopigmented dots. These wounds, when they heal, might not induce activation and migration of melanocytes to restore normal skin color. This is most evident in patients with darker complexions. On rare occasions there may be hyperpigmentation.

Folliculitis

Occasionally, a folliculitis may occur at the donor site. This may be secondary to hair spicules that are left behind in the skin or partially transected hairs trying to grow through the healed donor sites. Treatment with warm soaks and opening of any pustules can be helpful. On occasion the use of suitable antibiotics may speed recovery. If an infection is suspected in the area, a culture and sensitivity study may be appropriate.

DISCUSSION

The use of a robotic device to perform FUE-type hair transplantation is an important innovation in hair restoration. The machine is in itself a remarkable technical achievement combining a computer interface, imaging analysis, and a robotic arm.

For patients, the attraction to this type of a procedure is severalfold. The process is considered to be less invasive than strip harvesting and does not involve the creation of a linear scar. There may be quicker healing and the patient may have an earlier resumption of strenuous activities compared with strip harvesting. Compared with manual FUE, robotic harvesting is often more consistent and generally more rapid while still maintaining acceptable levels of transection.

From the authors' perspective, the ideal candidates for the robotic procedure or simply FUE/FIT include young patients who have not had prior harvesting and need a relatively small amount of grafts. Such patients can then have a greater chance of wearing their hair quite short if they decide not to proceed with further grafting. Other candidates include those people averse to the concept of strip excision and those with tight scalps that preclude strip harvesting.

For physicians desiring to include hair restoration procedures in their practice or for those who want to add FUE to an existing "strip" practice, the robot solves some of the key issues involved in learning how to perform the procedure. With proper instruction the physician can produce a reasonable number of grafts in a short time and achieve acceptable levels of transection. The robotic system also allows the physician to perform hair transplantation with a limited staff.

For those who adopt the robotic system early on, there is a perception that such doctors are in the vanguard. Whether that is true or not there may be marketing appeal coincident with having the device. Tangential to this point is that the FUE process, whether done with a manual technique or with a drill or the robotic system, is sometimes marketed as a procedure that allows the patient to wear his hair at any length. Such statements are false and misleading. When a significant number of grafts are harvested, if the scalp is shaved, the scars from the procedure are obvious to the naked eye.

It should be evident that the robotic system is not the perfect answer for all hair transplantation efforts. There are shortcomings and these are essentially similar to those encountered in FUE. A prominent concern is the thinning of the donor area with continued harvesting and the appearance of hypopigmented scars if the hair is cut too short.

Importantly, the use of the robotic machine does not eliminate the need for the physician to be able to diagnose male-pattern hair loss and other hair disorders. The physician must still learn the aesthetic aspects of the hair restoration process and how to approach various levels of hair loss to achieve successful outcomes.

It is the authors' opinion that it behooves the physician to know how to perform manual FUE/FIT and strip harvesting in the instance that there is an intraoperative need to abandon the robotic procedure.

The authors urge anyone unfamiliar with hair restoration, who desires to perform hair restoration surgery, to learn about the various aspect of hair loss diagnosis and treatment and seek appropriate training. The International Society of Hair Restoration Surgery (www.ishrs.org) is an excellent source and the society offers numerous courses around the world.

REFERENCES

1. Rassman W, Bernstein R, Szaniawski W, et al. Follicular transplantation. Int J Aesthet Restor Surg 1995;3:119–32.
2. Headington JT. Transverse microscopic anatomy of the human scalp. A basis for a morphometric approach to disorders of the hair follicle. Arch Dermatol 1984;120(4):449–56.
3. Orentreich N. Autografts in alopecias and other selected dermatologic conditions. Ann N Y Acad Sci 1959;83:463–79.
4. Rassman WR, Harris JA, Bernstein RM. Follicular unit extraction. In: Haber RS, Stough DB, editors. Hair transplantation. Philadelphia: Elsevier Saunders; 2006. p. 139–42.
5. Rassman W, Bernstein R, McClellan R, et al. Follicular Unit Extraction: minimally invasive surgery for hair transplantation. Dermatol Surg 2002;28:720–8.
6. Rose P. Approach to FIT. Presented at the International Society of Hair Restoration Surgery. Sydney (Australia), August 18–22, 2005.
7. Berman DA. New computer assisted system may change the hair restoration field. Practical Dermatology 2011;32–5.
8. Cole J. Body to scalp, donor area harvesting. In: Unger W, Shapiro R, Unger R, et al, editors. Hair transplantation. 5th edition. New York: Informa Healthcare; 2011. p. 304–6.
9. Harris JA. New methodology and instrumentation for follicular unit extraction: lower follicle transection rates and expanded patient candidacy. Dermatol Surg 2006;32:56–62.
10. Onda M, Igawa HH, Inoue K, et al. Novel technique of follicular unit hair transplantation with a powered punching device. Dermatol Surg 2008; 34:1683–8.
11. Winnington P. Robotic surgery: with new technology come new opportunities? Practical Dermatology 2012;1–2.
12. Canales M. Robotic hair transplantation: experience and results of first human clinical testing.

Presentation at the ISHRS Annual Meeting. Las Vegas (NV), September 26–30, 2007.

13. Rose P. The latest innovations in hair transplantation. Facial Plast Surg 2011;27(4):366–77.

14. Harris JA. Robotic assisted follicular unit extraction for hair restoration: case reports. Cosmet Dermatol 2012;25(6):284–7.

15. Vandruff CL. Artas System: how technology is changing the hair restoration industry. Aesthetic Trends 2011;1–5.

16. Unger W. The donor area harvesting. In: Unger W, Shapiro R, Unger R, et al, editors. Hair transplantation. 5th edition. New York: Informa Healthcare; 2011. p. 257–8.

17. Rose P. Logistics of FIT. Presented at the European Society of Hair Restoration Surgery meeting. Brussels, Belgium, June 2–5, 2005.

18. Rose P. FIT, problems, solutions and complications. Presented at the Orlando Live Surgery Workshop, Orlando (FL), March 3–6, 2005.

Index

Note: Page numbers of article titles are in **boldface** type.

A

ACD. *See* Allergic contact dermatitis (ACD)
Allergen(s)
  cosmetic-induced
    CAPB, 6
    common, 4–7
    fragrances, 5
    gallates, 6
    GMT, 6
    Myroxylon pereirae, 5
    patch testing for, 6–7
    PPD, 6
    preservatives, 4
    TSFR, 6
Allergic contact dermatitis (ACD)
  cosmetic-induced, **1–11**
    of anogenital area, 4
    common allergens, 4–7. *See also* Allergen(s),
      cosmetic-induced
    epidemiology of, 2
    evaluation of, 2
    of eyelids, 3
    of face, 2–3
    of hands, 3–4
    introduction, 1–2
    management of, 7–8
    of neck, 3
    of scalp, 4
Aluma
  in radiofrequency in cosmetic dermatology, 87–88
Anogenital area
  cosmetic-induced ACD of, 4
Apocrine gland, 65

B

Bipolar delivery
  of radiofrequency in cosmetic dermatology, 81
Bipolar devices
  in radiofrequency in cosmetic dermatology, 87–88
    Aluma, 87–88
    eMatrix, 88
BoNT. *See* Botulinum toxin (BoNT)
Botulinum toxin (BoNT), **23–36**
  adverse effects of, 26
  aesthetic uses of, 28–32
    bunny lines, 30
    chemical browlift, 29
    dimpled chin, 31
    forehead wrinkles, 29
    future directions in, 32–33
    glabellar lines, 28–29
    gummy smile, 30–31
    marionette lines, 31
    masseter hypertrophy, 32
    perioral lines, 31
    periorbital lines, 30
    platysmal bands, 32
  background of, 23
  contraindications to, 26
  conversion ratios, 27
  diffusion of, 28
  formulations of
    noninterchangeability of, 25–26
  handling and storage of, 26–27
  history of, 23–24
  immunogenicity of, 26
  mechanism of action of, 24–25
  in medical terminology, 32
  onset and duration of, 27
  structure of, 24–25
Browlift
  chemical
    BoNT for, 29
Bunny lines
  BoNT for, 30

C

Cancer(s)
  skin
    diagnosis of
      cutaneous laser surgery in, 65–66
CAPB. *See* Cocamidopropyl betaine (CAPB)
Carrier peptides, 16
Cellulite, **51–59**
  anatomy of, 51–52
  grading of, 52–53
  introduction, 51
  treatment of, **51–59**
    baseline photography in, 53
    complications in, 57
    long-term recommendations in, 58
    nonpharmacologic, 54–55
    outcome of
      evaluation of, 58
    pharmacologic, 54
    resistance to, 57
    surgical, 55–57

Dermatol Clin 32 (2014) 109–112
http://dx.doi.org/10.1016/S0733-8635(13)00120-4
0733-8635/14/$ – see front matter © 2014 Elsevier Inc. All rights reserved.

Moving?

Make sure your subscription moves with you!

To notify us of your new address, find your **Clinics Account Number** (located on your mailing label above your name), and contact customer service at:

Email: journalscustomerservice-usa@elsevier.com

800-654-2452 (subscribers in the U.S. & Canada)
314-447-8871 (subscribers outside of the U.S. & Canada)

Fax number: 314-447-8029

Elsevier Health Sciences Division
Subscription Customer Service
3251 Riverport Lane
Maryland Heights, MO 63043

*To ensure uninterrupted delivery of your subscription, please notify us at least 4 weeks in advance of move.

Printed and bound by CPI Group (UK) Ltd, Croydon, CR0 4YY

03/10/2024

01040378-0010